The Blood Type

The complete Guide on How and What to Eat for Your Blood Type (B) Recipes and four-week meal plain for Healthy Living and General Wellness

By

Gerald V. Lu

Table of contents

Introduction

FOOD HAS THE potential to heal and strengthen our physical bodies, support our recovery from injury and illness, and potentially change our genetic destinies.

Not only does food provide sustenance and nourishment, it provides an opportunity for creative expression and community, whether through developing new recipes or ways to prepare a certain food or in sharing a meal with others.

When I wrote Eat Right 4 Your Type in 1996, I explored the connections between blood type and diet, and outlined specific nutritional programs for each blood type. Since its publication more than fifteen years ago, I have continued to research and write about the role that foods play in our lives, and I have tried to create support materials and guidance for people who follow the Blood Type Diet.

In 1998, I wrote Cook Right 4 Your Type, which acted as a handbook for my readers, providing recipes, cooking tips, and planning guidelines to help navigate the process of food planning and preparation. I always wanted to take this further as I felt there was an aesthetic quality about food and food preparation that should be reflected in a book, not just with great recipes but also with beautiful, four-color photography that celebrates food. About three years ago, I met Kristin O'Connor. Although she came to see me as a patient, our conversation turned to following the Blood Type Diet, cooking, food preparation, and the work she was doing as a personal chef, food stylist, and food blogger.

I was impressed by her dedication to nutrition and healthy eating and by her ability to simplify the food-preparation process, which for some people can be quite daunting. Over the ensuing months, as we worked together as doctor and patient, our conversations returned again and again to food. I felt that I had found in Kristin the perfect person to collaborate on a book project that would blend the scientific concepts of the Blood Type Diet with the artistry of cooking to create visually stunning cookbooks specifically designed for each blood type. Kristin has a passion for the Blood Type Diet that is unparalleled, and an encyclopedic knowledge of the food lists for each of the blood types. She is creative and resourceful, and she appreciates and respects the need for food to both taste delicious and be nourishing.

For the past year, I have been enjoying the recipes included in the books, and I have to say that I've been knocked out by how delicious they are. They are also easy to prepare, as I know most of us have limited hours in the day for food planning and preparation. The recipes contained in these books are suitable for individuals or families, as well as for special events and entertaining.

Additionally, there are helpful food preparation tips, suggestions for how to organize your kitchen, food storage guidelines, and suggested resources that can make meal planning and preparation easier. My goal has always been to provide accessible information that is easy to incorporate into daily life, and I believe that Kristin has accomplished this.

These cookbooks represent new food and healthy lifestyle possibilities for my readers; they combine the science behind the Blood Type Diet with Kristin's expertise not only as a chef but as a believer and follower of these concepts, and package them in a beautiful, four-color format. The recipes contained within are appropriate for your blood type and compliant with the food lists, and they are delicious and made with love—love of food, love of health, and love of sharing this with others on both Kristin's and my part.

I invite you to join us on the continued journey of personalized living. I am confident that you will find a trusted companion in these cookbooks, and one who will make your life richer and healthier as you experiment with the recipes that were developed specifically to be right for your type.

IN THE BLOOD-TYPE world, B stands for Balance. To be as healthy as possible, Type B should not only strive for balance in their meals, but also in life. As Type As achieve health through a mostly vegetarian diet and Type O should maintain a protein-rich, carnivorous diet, Type B works best by enjoying the best of both worlds. Whereas with the other blood types there are large groups of foods to avoid, Type B has highly Beneficial foods in every category: meats, grains, dairy, fruits, and vegetables. Type B has a wide array of cheeses to select from, not to mention three Neutrals that are on most blood types' Avoid list: beer, red wine, and coffee...lucky you. Of course, Neutrals are not going to improve your health, but in moderation they won't harm you either. Let's briefly review what it means to be a Type B.

When structuring meals for the day, Type Bs should try to have a protein, complex carbohydrate, and vegetable with each dish. Protein is best achieved through red meats such as lamb, mutton, and rabbit as well as a variety of cheeses, beans, and an abundant selection of seafood. Chicken, shellfish, and soy proteins should be avoided. Between the selection of Beneficial and Neutral grains, there is not much to avoid besides corn. You will have ample choice between many delicious grains, breads, and pastas. Fruits and vegetable options are also plentiful, just be sure to avoid tomatoes.

Type Bs are fortunate to be known for their strong immune systems, aiding in their ability to be adaptable to various dietary and environmental influences. It's for this reason that Type Bs should eat a diverse and balanced diet. Disease susceptibility in Type B occurs when there are imbalances in the body, typically resulting in autoimmune disease or rare, slow-growing viruses. Type Bs are also at risk for Type I diabetes and chronic fatigue syndrome. Maintaining a balanced diet and adhering to Type B Beneficials, however, will help prevent these medical risks.

The Blood Type Diet has taken personalized nutrition to a higher level with

the introduction of the influence Secretor Status has on our health. Approximately 80 percent of the population are Secretors, which means that the majority of us secrete our blood-type antigens in our bodily fluids such as saliva and mucus. As I wrote in Live Right 4 Your Type:

Subtyping your blood, especially your Secretor Status, provides an even greater specificity of identification. Your blood type doesn't just sit inert in your body. It is expressed in countless ways...A simple analogy would be a faucet. Depending on the water pressure, the faucet might pour or dribble...In the same way, your Secretor Status relates to how much and where your blood type antigen is expressed in your body.

Being a Secretor means that we can immediately attack viruses, bacteria, and other foreign bodies as they come in contact with our bodies, through secretions in our saliva. Non-Secretors do not have this first line of defense; however, their internal defenses are more powerful than Secretors. All of this means that some foods that are suitable for Secretors may not be for Non-Secretors (NS), and vice versa. To address this, we have tagged all recipes in this book that are appropriate for Non-Secretors, and when possible, substitutions are provided to make the other recipes acceptable and healthful for Non-Secretors.

Just as your food should be balanced, so should your exercise regimen. The most effective workout strategies for your blood type are those that balance moderate physical exertion with a mental component, so stick to hiking, biking, tennis, and swimming, most of which are also gentle on the knees.

In this book, you will find recipes, menus, and tools specifically designed for your Type B diet and Secretor Status. For more information, see Eat Right 4 Your Type, the Blood Type B Food, Beverage and Supplement Lists, or refer to

your SWAMI© Personalized Nutrition Software Program guide if you have one (SWAMI is a proprietary software program designed to produce a unique, one- of-a-kind diet protocol based on your blood type, a series of biometric measurements and your personal history. See page 236 in the Appendix).

Type B is the adventurous blood type, encouraged to explore and try new things. Type B has the luxury of eating all kinds of interesting foods and eating them in combination with one another, so don't be afraid to dig in and get started on your own blood-type adventure.

Chapter 1: Type Food list

Here is a list of basics to keep in your kitchen with the thought that there will be times when meals have to be spontaneous. If you have essentials from your Beneficial and Neutral lists on hand, no matter what you make, it will be something good for you.

Salad Base

Pick your favorite greens or mix it up each time you go to the grocery store, keeping these salad-base options in mind:

BENEFICIALS

Cabbage Kale

NEUTRALS

Arugula Boston Bibb Escarole

Red-leaf lettuce Spinach

These will give you a great start to a last-minute salad or an added crunch to a sandwich.

Roasted Vegetables

The best thing you could do for yourself is to keep hearty fresh vegetables on hand. They are perfect to roast for dinner, make in bulk to add to your last- minute salad the next day, or throw in a frittata for breakfast. Roasted vegetables are a terrific leftover to keep on hand. Most vegetables work well when tossed with olive oil, sea salt, and roasted in a 375-degree oven for 12 to 20 minutes (depending on the size and density of the vegetables.) Here are a few that are both Beneficial to Type B and take well to roasting:

BENEFICIALS

Beets Broccoli Carrots Cauliflower Eggplant Kale Parsnips Peppers

Sweet potatoes/yams Turnips

NEUTRALS

Asparagus Celeriac Fennel Onions Potatoes Squash Zucchini

Keeping a few of these vegetables in your fridge each week will come in handy and is a perfect way to add more Beneficials to your diet.

Fruit

Most people don't have a problem incorporating fruit in their diet. It is a perfect snack, paired with nuts or nut butters, used to make desserts, and added to cereal or salads. Some fruits even work well in savory dishes. Below is a list of Beneficial fruit for Type B:

BENEFICIALS

Bananas Cranberries Grapes Papayas Pineapples Plums Watermelon

Milk

Type Bs are among the few who benefit from cow's milk, which is a great source of protein. The best milk options for Type Bs are: Nonfat or 2 percent cow's milk

Protein

The Type B diet is based on balanced protein and vegetable consumption, so it is important to keep a diverse supply of proteins to accompany vegetables and grains at each meal. We suggest keeping two fresh types of proteins in the fridge and then two to three in the freezer for backup. Prepare more meat than you need and save the rest as leftovers to enjoy the next day for lunch or to add to a casserole. Here are a few staples that are useful to have on hand. Please note, it is recommended that all poultry be organic and all beef be grass-fed and organic.

BENEFICIALS

Cheeses (cottage cheese, farmer cheese, feta, goat cheese, kefir, mozzarella, ricotta) Lamb (cheaper and contain more lean meat than chops or rack) Nut butter (walnut butter made from black walnuts) Seafood (cod, flounder, grouper, halibut, mahimahi, salmon, sole)

NEUTRALS

Beef tips

Cheeses (Brie, Camembert, Cheddar, Colby, cream cheese, Gouda, Gruyere, Jarlsberg, Monterey Jack, Muenster, Parmesan, provolone, Swiss) Eggs

Ground beef (90 percent lean or leaner) Nut butters (almond, pecan, or macadamia. Almond butter is inexpensive and easily found in supermarkets or natural food stores.) Seafood (catfish, herring, orange roughy, red snapper, sole, squid, tilapia, whitefish) Turkey tenderloins

Filling up Your Freezer

Smoothies

Making smoothies is a great alternative for breakfast or a perfect protein-filled snack. They are a go-to recipe that you should be sure you have ingredients for at all times. Of course, fresh fruit can be used when in season. Mix in some frozen fruits and vegetables into the smoothie for a thicker consistency, however. Here are a few Beneficial options:

BENEFICIALS

Bananas Kale Pineapple

NEUTRALS

Figs Mangos Peaches Raspberries Strawberries

Leftovers

It's always helpful to double the recipe when making foods that freeze easily such as: Chili

Cookies Crackers Lasagna Muffins Pesto Sauces Stews

Pesto can be stored in BPA-free ice cube trays for individual servings. On the following pages, you will find more information on safe food storage as well as suggestions for cooking in bulk.

Protein

Just like keeping fresh protein options in your fridge, it is always helpful to keep at least a few in the freezer as well. To defrost meats, poultry, or seafood, take them out the day before and put them in the refrigerator. It is recommended that all beef be grass fed and organic.

BENEFICIALS

Beef tips

Ground beef (90 percent lean or leaner) Lamb steaks (cheaper and contain more lean meat than chops or rack) Turkey (ground, tenderloins, whole) Seafood (cod, flounder, grouper, halibut, mahimahi, salmon, sole)

NEUTRALS

Seafood (catfish, herring, orange roughy, red snapper, scallops, squid, tilapia, whitefish)

Time to Get in That Pantry

Snacks

The first thing we all go into the pantry for is to grab a quick bite on the run or pack a snack to ship off to school with the kids. It's pretty important that these midday treats are balanced and wholesome; the best way to make that happen is to stock that pantry right. Here are a few staples for Type Bs: Almond butter

Brown rice cakes

Dark chocolate (70 percent or higher) Dried fruit (banana chips, cranberries, figs, prunes) Fresh fruit (bananas, grapes, papaya, pineapple, plums, watermelon) Nuts (almonds, pecans, macadamia nuts, walnuts) Spelt crackers

Whole-grain cereals (made from oat, spelt, or brown rice)

If you want to prep ahead for those times when you are in a rush, mix combinations of nuts, dried fruit, and maybe even a little dark chocolate, and divide into single servings. Store in small glass sealable containers and take them in the car, on the plane, or anywhere you are headed.

Drinks

Drinking water is always the best option, but when you want to add a little flavor to your beverage repertoire, dabble in these Beneficial teas or Neutral drinks, but try not to go overboard with Neutrals. There are a few drink recipes in this book.

BENEFICIALS

Grape juice Pineappale juice

Teas (ginger, green, licorice, peppermint, rose hip)

NEUTRALS

Beer Black tea Coffee Red wine

Grains/Legumes

Grains should be an integral part of the Type B diet, eaten in balance with protein and vegetables at each meal. There are quite a few grains to choose from, which are both Beneficial and Neutral and will add variety to any meal.

Quinoa, for example, cooks in 12 minutes and is a light but filling side for a fast weeknight dinner. Beans are also a perfect way to add satiating proteins and carbohydrates to salads, casseroles, stews, dips, and soups.

Beans (kidney, lima, navy)

Whole grains (millet, oat bran, oat meal, puffed rice, rice bran, rice cakes, spelt)

Seasonings

Making healthy food taste good is non-negotiable. One quick trick to doing so is by knowing your way around your spice cabinet. Herbs and spices are calorie free and flavor packed. The spices listed below also happen to be terrific for your Type B body. Keep a jar of homemade bread crumbs on hand for a quick topping on a casserole, used as turkey breading, or to bread seafood.

Additionally, as much as we would like to repress our sweet tooth, it is an unrealistic expectation for most, so stock up on natural sweeteners like agave and maple syrup, although try to use sparingly.

BENEFICIALS

Basic Bread Crumbs   Olive oil

Molasses

Spices (cayenne pepper, curry, ginger, horseradish, parsley)

NEUTRALS

Spices (anise, basil, bay leaf, caraway, cardamom, carob, chili powder, chive, clove, coriander, cumin, garlic, marjoram, mustard, nutmeg, oregano, paprika, red pepper flakes, peppermint, sage, tamari, tamarind, tarragon, thyme, turmeric, vanilla) Maple syrup

Agave nectar Vinegar

Recipe Ideas for Last-Minute Cooking

Time-Saving Tricks

Make these recipes in bulk and store in your freezer to grab on the go: flax chips, smoothies in individual portions, baked goods, chili, granola, soups, casseroles, pesto in ice-cube trays, or stews.

When making dressings or condiments, double or triple the recipe and store it in the refrigerator for future use. If you are making a recipe that uses one lemon, you might as well do it with three and save yourself the prep and clean- up again and again.

Utilize Roasted Vegetables

Let's reemphasize here how amazingly useful leftover roasted vegetables can be. Not only are they ready to be thrown into just about any savory dish, but they add tremendous flavor with no effort whatsoever. Here are a few examples where you can toss in roasted vegetables and have a tasty new dish: Casseroles

Cold pasta salad Crêpes

Frittata Lettuce wraps Omelets Pizza Quiches

Rice Salads Soufflés

Spring rolls Taco salads Vegetable tarts

Next time you make roasted vegetables for dinner, do yourself a favor and double up on that recipe.

Review Your Stock

Now that you have the basics, it's time to take a look at some of the Avoids. You have lived your whole life eating whatever you want. Now you open your cabinets and think, how do I start over? but the answer is simple: you don't have to. You just have to emphasize the healthy choices that you are now privy to.

You should ditch anything that is categorized Best Avoided for your type; listed below are a few places where Avoids may be lurking and ready to sabotage your otherwise perfect, new diet.

Open up the fridge—take inventory of all condiments, sauces, stocks, and other processed foods.

Open the pantry—familiarize yourself with the ingredients in your snacks, cereals, pastas, spices, and other foods.

Open the freezer—remove frozen dinners. Just do it. You can be sure they are not doing you any good. Other than that, the same applies here as above: evaluate what you have, and review ingredients just to get yourself acquainted with what you are dealing with.

Once you have done that, take out all questionable subjects and line them up on the counter or table. Refer to the Type B diet in Eat Right 4 Your Type, the Blood Type B Food, Beverage, and Supplement List, or refer to your SWAMI personalized nutrition report food lists. Check out your Avoids, as this will be the most efficient way of eliminating those foods that are best Avoided.

Please note that Avoids are not limited to the examples listed below. Here is a rundown of the main offenders:

Corn

Corn has become a hot topic in the food world. The movie Food Inc. helped explain to many people that the mass production of corn has become a national, if not global, issue. With the introduction of genetically modified organisms (GMOs) or foods that are genetically altered to optimize their growing potential, corn quite literally became another species. As an Avoid for Type B, eliminating corn gives us yet another opportunity to clean our diet. Due to our society's dependence on corn, it is used in a wide range of processed goods, making it virtually impossible to avoid altogether.

We will do our best to outline where corn is generally hidden, but know, too, that with this diet, it is ok to run into an Avoid once in a while without sabotaging your progress. If you are not acutely sick and are simply using the Blood Type Diet for general health, you only have to be 80 percent compliant to see 100 percent results. How forgiving is that?

The following are a few places corn exists: Alcohol (some) Artificial flavorings

Artificial sweeteners Ascorbic acid Aspartame

Baked goods (some) Baking powder (some)

Canned fruits and some vegetables Caramel color Cereal

Cheese spreads Citric acid Confectioners' sugar Corn flour

Corn starch Corn syrup Food starch Grits Hominy

Hydrolyzed vegetable protein Ice cream (some)

Instant coffee/teas Ketchup

Licorice

Maize Malt/malt syrup

Modified food starch Molasses (some) Polenta

Popcorn

Prepared mustard (some) Salad dressings

Salt (iodized) Soda Splenda Sucrose

Sugar (if not cane or beet)

Sweet beverages (containing corn syrup) Taco shells Tomato sauce (with corn syrup)

Vitamins (some) Xanthan gum Yeast (some)

Yogurt (with corn syrup)

Soy

When most people hear they have to avoid soy, they say, "No problem, I can't stand tofu anyway." Unfortunately, soy is not only found in obvious places like soy sauce, tofu, or soy cheese. Due to its perceived adaptability, soy is used as a blank canvas to adapt to any flavor or texture. It is relatively inexpensive to produce, and it can be found in almost all processed foods today. The good news is, avoiding soy means avoiding most packaged foods that probably contain many ingredients that are unhealthy for you, so try to think of it as a great reminder to eat whole, pure foods as often as possible. Below is a list of foods that generally contain soy or are soy-based products. It is important to read food labels to make sure you are totally avoiding soy.

Artificial or natural flavors Canned tuna (some) Chocolate

Crisco Edamame

Fermented bean paste Gravy (some)

Hydrolyzed vegetable protein Mayonnaise

Miso

Mono-diglyceride Monosodium glutamate Salad dressings

Soy cheese Soy flour Soy milk Soy oil Soy sauce

Store-bought baked goods (some) Store-bought broth (some)

Soups (some)

Spice blends (some) Tamari

Tempeh Teriyaki sauce

Textured vegetable protein Tofu

Whipped toppings Worcestershire sauce

Wheat

Although Type Bs do not have to be gluten-free, it is beneficial for you to be as wheat free as possible, both for optimal weight loss and health. Luckily for you, there are plenty of non-wheat options to cook with and to buy as healthier substitutions. Spelt or brown rice breads are readily available in health food stores and online, and they are very close to the texture and taste of wheat breads.

Here are a few places where wheat exists: Baking powder (some) Beer Blue cheese (some)

Bread crumbs Breaded fish Breads Brewer's yeast Broth (some) Bulgur Candies (some)

Caramel color (some) Cereal

Chewing gum Cold cuts (some) Cookies Cornbread Couscous Crackers Croutons Dumplings Farina

Flavored extracts (some)

Food starch or modified food starch (some) Graham flour Gravy

Hot dogs Hush puppies

Hydrolyzed plant protein Hydrolyzed vegetable protein Ice cream (some)

Kamut

Malt (flavoring, and vinegar)

Matzo Meat loaf Meatballs

"Natural flavor" (either soy or gluten) Pancakes Pasta (including orzo)

Pastries Pie crust Pita bread Pizza crust

Potato chips (some) Pretzels

Salad dressings Seitan Semolina Soups

Soy sauce

Spice mixtures (some) Syrup

Tamari Teriyaki sauce

Textured vegetable protein Waffles

Wheat

Wheat protein Wheatgrass Worcestershire sauce

Chicken

Chicken seems to be the most difficult exclusion for Type Bs. The most challenging part of no longer eating chicken is figuring out options when eating out, because in your own kitchen it can easily be replaced with turkey in most recipes. Because Type Bs are made to have balanced diets, however, you can see that there are many options still available when dining out.

The Rest

Other than corn, soy, wheat, and chicken, it will be straightforward to determine what else to take out of your cabinets, fridge, and freezer. Take the time to go through your list of Avoids and remove them from your house. If you have canned goods, and nonperishables, you can donate to your local food bank. To find a food bank in your area, go to http://feedingamerica.org.

You should be all cleared out now, so you are ready to go to the store and grab a few essentials to fill in the gaps.

How to Read These Recipes

This cookbook is designed to be as practical and helpful to the Blood Type dieter as possible. We took into consideration that many families could be cooking for multiple blood types or preparing meals for friends with varying blood types. In order to make doing so practical, each of the Eat Right 4 Your Type Personalized Cookbooks contains the same or similar recipe ideas with different executions to suit the needs of each blood type. You will find the recipe titles almost identical in each book; however, ingredients and methods might vary quite a bit. There are many recipes that are Beneficial across the board and are marked with an (A/B/AB/O) to identify that they are universal to every type. For example, every blood type has a pancake recipe; however, Type Bs have Beneficial grains that might be on the Avoid list for other types, so each recipe contains different flours.

Every recipe is also written to contain as many Beneficial foods as possible with the understanding that taste is still of the utmost importance. After all, you are not going to be inclined to dive into a kale cookie, but you won't be able to resist Pasta Carbonara with Crispy Kale. The point is that we want you coming back for more each time to see that eating right for your blood type is as far from sacrifice as is indulging in a bar of chocolate.

As you make your way through this book, you will notice that once in a while there is a highlighted section called "Featured Ingredient." There are several ingredients used in this book that you may not have come across before, some that are Beneficial for your diet and some that are Beneficial for your taste buds. In an effort to familiarize you with these ingredients, there is a brief summary explaining a little about what that ingredient is, and how or why it is used. Don't be afraid to experiment with unfamiliar territory.

Many people who follow the Blood Type Diet come to my office or have used the tests on my website (www.dadamo.com) to create a specific diet plan for themselves. If you have done that, you have a SWAMI personalized nutrition report that may vary slightly from the general Type B diet because it takes into consideration family and medical history, Secretor Status, and GenoType. (The GenoType is a further refinement of my work in personalized nutrition. It uses a variety of simple measurements, combined with blood type data, to classify individuals as one of six basic Epigenotypes: The Hunter, Gatherer, Teacher, Explorer, Warrior, and Nomad types.). Due to the variations in Beneficial, Neutral, and Best Avoided foods, there may be some recipes containing ingredients that do not suit you as an individual. Please do not skip these recipes entirely. There is always a way to make quick and easy substitutions. (See

"Useful Tools: Substitutions," page 215.) As a quick piece of advice, however, vegetables can be easily swapped out—leafy greens for other leafy greens, a specific type of beans for another, or in some cases, simply omitted from the recipe if they are not a star component.

You will see that recipes are also tagged according to Secretor Status. Some recipes are not appropriate for Non-Secretors, but are fine for Secretors (see recipe legend below) in most instances. When this is the case, there are simple substitutions to adapt the recipe for Non-Secretors. In a few cases, however, the recipe will be an Avoid altogether for a Type B Non-Secretor.

In many of the recipes in this book, you will see sea salt written as "sea salt, to taste," and might be wondering what that means or how much to add. Salt can make or break your dish, but if you add too much, there is no going back. Try adding a little at a time, taste, and add more if needed. What is a little? Well, start with pinching a bit between your fingers and sprinkling it into your dish, give it a minute to incorporate, and then taste. If you were to measure a pinch, it would be a little less than 1/8 of a teaspoon.

Remember to read each recipe in its entirety before starting to ensure you know how much time it will take and if there are any ingredients you will need to buy ahead of time. Finally, enjoy making, eating, and sharing these recipes.

RECIPE LEGEND:

An * is used when a recipe ingredient needs further instruction, substitution, or comment. This information is found at the bottom of a recipe.

All recipes are appropriate for Type B Secretors.

 represents a recipe that is appropriate for Type B Non-Secretors. Recipe ingredients that are NOT appropriate for Type B Non-Secretors are notated with appropriate acceptable substitutions within recipe ingredients.

A REVIEW OF THE FOOD LISTS:

Throughout this book we refer to a number of places to find the comprehensive foods lists for the Blood Type Diet. Here's a recap of where you can find the lists so you can use the one that is right for you:

Eat Right 4 Your Type, which provides the entry point into the Blood Type Diet

Live Right 4 Your Type, which incorporates the value of the Secretor Status Blood Type B Food, Beverage, and Supplement Lists from Eat Right 4 Your Type, a handy pocket guide with the basic food lists

Change Your Genetic Destiny (originally published as The GenoType Diet, which provides a further refinement of the diet by using blood type, secretor status, and a series of biometric measurements to further individualize your food lists)

SWAMI Personalized Nutrition Software, designed to harness the power of computers and artificial intelligence, using their tremendous precision and speed to help tailor unique, one-of-a-kind diets. From its extensive knowledge base, SWAMI can evaluate more than 700 foods for more than 200 individual attributes (such as cholesterol level, gluten content, presence of antioxidants, etc.) to determine if that food is either a superfood or toxin for you. It provides a specific, unique diet in an easy-to-read, user-friendly format, complete with food lists, recipes, and meal planning.

Chapter 2: Breakfast

reakfast recipes were written with diversity in mind, so that you do not end up eating the same thing every day. The idea here is to alternate: one day

eggs, the next quinoa or granola, and so on, in order to keep providing your body with different nutrients each day. You will probably notice that the biggest change in these recipes is the types of flour used. Don't be intimidated; try one simple recipe like pancakes to get your feet wet and move on to the rest. Once you have the new flour on hand, the rest is just like any other recipe.

1/2 cup quinoa

1/2 cup water

1/ cup 2 percent cow's milk

1/ teaspoon sea salt

2 tablespoons dried cherries

1 tablespoon dried cranberries 2 tablespoons slivered almonds 2 tablespoons chopped walnuts 2 teaspoons maple syrup

1/ cup crunchy rice cereal

1.   Rinse quinoa. Combine in a small saucepan with water, milk, salt, cherries, and cranberries, and bring to a boil. Cook 10 minutes, turn off the heat, and let sit an additional 4 to 5 minutes. Quinoa will absorb all the water and become light and fluffy when done.

2.   While the quinoa cooks, toast almonds and walnuts in a dry skillet for about 2 minutes or until slightly golden brown. Watch nuts carefully; because of their high fat content, they have a tendency to burn easily.

3.   Fluff cooked quinoa with a fork and add toasted nuts and maple syrup. Top with crunchy rice cereal and add more milk if desired.

4.   Serve immediately.

SERVES 2

4 cups crispy rice cereal 1 cup chopped walnuts 1 cup chopped pecans

1/4 cup halved whole flaxseeds

1/4 cup blackstrap molasses 2 teaspoons olive oil

1 tablespoon agave 1/8 teaspoon sea salt 1/4 cup water

1 cup halved dried cherries

1/2 cup dried cranberries

1.   Preheat oven to 350 degrees. Line a sheet pan with parchment paper and set aside.

2.   In a large bowl, combine rice cereal, walnuts, pecans, and flaxseeds. Set aside.

3.   In a small saucepan, warm molasses, olive oil, agave, and salt with water over medium heat for about 2 minutes, whisking to combine.

4.   Pour molasses mixture over granola mixture, toss to coat, and spread onto prepared sheet pan. Bake 10 minutes. Reduce oven temperature to 300 degrees.

5.   Take granola out of the oven, toss, and place back in the oven. Bake an additional 25 minutes.

6.   Toss with cherries and cranberries.

7.   Serve warm or cool fully, and store in an airtight, glass container for up to 2 weeks or in the freezer for up to 2 months.

MAKES 32 (1/2-CUP) SERVINGS

3 tablespoons walnut or almond butter

1/ cup granola* Sea salt, to taste 2 bananas

1.   Stir nut butter, granola, and salt until granola is evenly coated.

2.   Peel bananas, and slice in half down the center and then in half lengthwise, so you have 4 long pieces of banana. Spoon 2 teaspoons granola mixture on each piece of banana and enjoy.

SERVES 2

egg salad:

2 teaspoons olive oil

1/ cup cooked or canned kidney beans, drained and rinsed 3 hardboiled eggs

1/ cup mozzarella cheese

1 tablespoon chopped parsley 2 cups mixed baby greens Sea salt, to taste

dressing:

1/ teaspoon mustard powder 1 tablespoon olive oil

1 tablespoon lemon juice 1 tablespoon onion, grated Sea salt, to taste

1.   In a small skillet, heat olive oil over medium heat. Toast kidney beans 2 to 3 minutes until warm and slightly crunchy. Set aside.

2.   Remove eggs from shells, and use a fork to break apart in a bowl. Set aside. In a separate bowl, whisk together all dressing ingredients. Pour over eggs and toss.

3.   Add beans, cheese, and parsley to eggs, and toss. Serve over mixed baby greens.

SERVES 4

Nonstick cooking spray 3 strips turkey bacon

3 large whole eggs

3 large egg whites

2 teaspoons olive oil 2 cups fresh spinach Sea salt, to taste

1/ cup mozzarella cheese

4 slices brown rice/ millet or spelt toast

1.   Heat a large skillet over medium heat, and coat with nonstick cooking spray.

2.   Add bacon and cook 3 to 4 minutes, flip, and cook an additional 2 to 3 minutes on the opposite side for crispy bacon. Remove from pan, let cool, then crumble and set aside.

3.   Whisk eggs and egg whites in a small bowl. Set aside. In the same skillet, add olive oil and reduce heat slightly. Add spinach, sauté 2 minutes, and season mixture with sea salt to taste. Pour eggs over spinach, cooking gently until done, about 2 minutes. Turn off heat and add reserved bacon and cheese.

4.   Spoon mixture on toast and serve immediately.

SERVES 4

tip: If the bacon is not as crispy as you like, you can add a drizzle of olive oil to help it along.

2 teaspoons ghee 1/4 cup finely diced Spanish onion

1 cup diced cremini mushrooms 3 cups chopped Swiss chard

3 large whole eggs

3 large egg whites

2 tablespoons spelt flour Sea salt, to taste

1 teaspoon chopped fresh tarragon 1 teaspoon olive oil

1.   Preheat oven to 375 degrees.

2.   Melt ghee in an ovenproof sauté pan over medium heat. Sauté onion, mushrooms, and Swiss chard for 4 to 5 minutes, until chard has wilted and vegetables are tender. Set aside.

3.   While onion mixture is cooking, whisk together eggs, egg whites, flour, salt, and tarragon in a large bowl. Add olive oil to skillet and pour egg mixture over vegetables. Cook for about 1 minute, just until set.

4.   Transfer pan to oven and bake 6 to 8 minutes, or until firm and edges are golden.

SERVES 4

1 head broccoli

1/ teaspoon sea salt

1   tablespoon plus 2 teaspoons olive oil, divided 3 large whole eggs

2   large egg whites

1/ cup crumbled feta

1/ cup chopped spinach

1/ cup finely diced chives

2 teaspoon brown rice or spelt flour 1 tablespoon chopped oregano

1.   Preheat oven to 375 degrees.

2.   Dice broccoli into bite-size pieces, place in a single layer on a baking sheet, and sprinkle with a dash of sea salt and 1 tablespoon olive oil. Bake 15 minutes.

3.   In a medium-size bowl, whisk eggs, egg whites, feta, spinach, chives, flour, oregano, and salt until well combined.

4.   Brush a medium-size, ovenproof skillet with remaining 2 teaspoons olive oil and heat over medium heat, to create a nonstick surface. Add egg mixture to hot pan with broccoli. Cook 1 to 2 minutes, lifting the side of the eggs gently with your spatula to encourage uncooked egg to run down into the bottom of the skillet.

5.   If the handle of your skillet is rubber, wrap tightly with tinfoil to prevent melting. Place skillet under the broiler for 2 minutes, or until the eggs set and brown very slightly on the edges.

6.   Serve warm.

SERVES 4

1/4 cup finely chopped white onion 3 cups chopped kale

1 cup diced zucchini

1/3 cup finely diced red bell peppers 4 teaspoons olive oil, divided

1/2 pound ground turkey sausage 1 tablespoon maple syrup

3 large eggs

2 large egg whites 1 tablespoon water

Large-grain sea salt, to taste

1/ cup diced kefir cheese

1.   In a large skillet, sauté onion, kale, zucchini, and peppers in 2 teaspoons olive oil over medium heat for 3 to 4 minutes, or until vegetables are aromatic and tender and kale is bright green and wilted. Remove from skillet and set aside.

2.   Brown turkey sausage in the same skillet with remaining 2 teaspoons olive oil over medium heat, breaking into bite-size pieces until cooked through, about 5 to 6 minutes. Drizzle with maple syrup, and stir to coat. Add sausage to vegetables and set aside.

3.   Return skillet to stovetop and reduce heat to medium-low. Whisk eggs and egg whites with water and salt to taste, and add to skillet. Stir gently with a heat- safe spatula until firm and cooked through. Add sausage and vegetables to the skillet, and stir to combine.

4.   Serve topped with kefir cheese.

SERVES 4

2 teaspoons olive oil

1/2 cup finely diced onion

1/2 cup finely diced fennel

1 pound ground turkey meat 1 teaspoon fennel seed

1   teaspoon paprika 1 teaspoon sea salt

1/4 teaspoon chili powder 1 clove garlic, minced

1/2 cup finely diced Bosc pear 2 teaspoons maple syrup

1.   In a large sauté pan, heat olive oil over medium heat. Add onions and fennel, and sauté 3 to 4 minutes, or until tender. Remove from heat and let cool to room temperature, about 10 minutes.

2.   Place ground turkey in a large bowl, and add fennel seed, paprika, salt, chili powder, garlic, pear, maple syrup, and cooled vegetables. Use your hands to incorporate all ingredients into the meat, but do not over mix.

3.   Form meat into small, hot dog–shaped links. Cook 8 to 10 minutes or until meat is browned on all sides and inside of the sausage is no longer pink.

4.   Serve warm alone or alongside scrambled eggs for a protein-packed breakfast.

SERVES 4

2   teaspoons olive oil, plus more for greasing 1 teaspoon ghee

2 cups diced onion

2 cups quartered white mushrooms 2 cups diced zucchini

6 cups torn kale Sea salt, to taste

8 cups (1-inch) bread cubes (sprouted wheat or spelt bread) 1 cup 2 percent cow's milk

1 cup Vegetable Stock* 4 large eggs, beaten

1 teaspoon fresh thyme

1 teaspoon fresh rosemary 1 teaspoon fresh sage

1 cup mozzarella cheese

1.   Preheat oven to 350 degrees. Grease a 9" x 11" baking dish with olive oil and set aside.

2.   In a large skillet, heat ghee and 2 teaspoons olive oil over medium heat. Sauté onion, mushrooms, zucchini, and kale until tender, about 5 to 6 minutes. Season with salt, and set aside.

3.   Spread bread cubes in a single layer on a baking sheet. Toast for 3 to 4 minutes, until slightly golden brown. Toss in a large bowl with vegetables.

4.   Whisk together milk, stock, eggs, thyme, rosemary, and sage. Pour over bread and vegetables, and toss to combine. Pour the entire mixture into the prepared baking dish. Top with mozzarella cheese and bake, covered, for 35 minutes. Uncover, and bake an additional 10 minutes, until cheese is bubbling and slightly browned.

5.   Serve warm.

SERVES 12

1   tablespoon ghee

2   tablespoons spelt or oat flour

1/2 cup 2 percent cow's milk

1/2 cup Vegetable Stock* 2 cups packed spinach

1 cup chopped red bell pepper 2 large egg yolks

1/4 cup chopped basil

1/4 cup grated Gruyere cheese 1/4 teaspoon cayenne pepper Sea salt, to taste

4 egg whites, at room temperature

1.   Preheat oven to 350 degrees. Spray 4 (12-oz.) ramekins with nonstick cooking spray, place in a baking dish, and set aside.

2.   In a saucepan over medium heat, melt ghee and whisk in flour. Gradually add milk and stock, whisking continuously until thickened, about 3 to 4 minutes. Once mixture is thick and resembles the consistency of yogurt, remove from the

heat and let cool completely.

3.   In a food processor, puree spinach and bell pepper. Place pureed vegetables onto cheesecloth or paper towels, wrap the cloth around the vegetables, and strain excess liquid by gently squeezing the vegetable juice through the cloth. Place vegetables in a bowl, and whisk in egg yolks, basil, cheese, cayenne, and salt. Set aside.

4.   Fold milk mixture into vegetable mixture and set aside.

5.   In a dry, glass bowl, beat egg whites with a hand mixer until they form stiff peaks. Fold the egg whites, one-third at a time, into the vegetables. Spoon mixture into prepared ramekins, and fill the baking dish halfway with hot water. Carefully place in the oven and bake for 45 minutes or until tester inserted into ramekin comes out clean.

6.   Serve immediately.

SERVES 4

1/ cup oat flour

1/ cup spelt flour

1/ teaspoon sea salt

11/ cups 2 percent cow's milk 2 large eggs

1   tablespoon plus 1 teaspoon melted ghee or butter, divided

1.   In a medium bowl, whisk flours and sea salt.

2.   Combine milk, eggs, and 1 tablespoon melted ghee, and beat well. Add to flour mixture, and whisk until well blended. Cover and place in the refrigerator for 1 hour.

3.   Heat a large sauté pan over medium heat. When the pan is hot, add remaining 1 teaspoon ghee and brush evenly across the bottom of the pan. Using a 1/ -cup measuring cup, scoop batter into pan and quickly turn the pan in circular motions to spread the batter into a very thin layer. Let cook 1 minute or until the batter firms and edges lift slightly off the pan. Use an offset spatula to flip and cook 1 additional minute.

SERVES 4

tip: For an indulgent treat, top with banana slices, walnuts, and Chocolate Syrup NS (page 209).

muffins:

2   cups spelt flour 1 cup oat flour

2 teaspoons baking powder

1/2 teaspoon baking soda

1/2 teaspoon fine-grain sea salt

1/8 teaspoon ground cloves

1/2 teaspoon ground ginger

1/ teaspoon allspice (NS omit allspice and add 1/ teaspoon nutmeg) 1 (15-oz.) can organic sweet potatoes

1/ cup honey

2 large eggs

1/ cup 2 percent cow's milk

topping:

1/ cup rolled oats

1/ cup finely chopped pecans 1 tablespoon honey

. 1   tablespoon almond or light olive oil

1/ cup Carob Extract™*

1.   Preheat oven to 350 degrees. Line a 12-cup muffin tin with paper liners and set aside.

2.   In a large bowl, stir together flours, baking powder, baking soda, salt, cloves, ginger, and allspice until well combined.

3.   In a separate bowl, whisk sweet potatoes, honey, eggs, and milk. Add the sweet potato mixture to the flour mixture and stir to incorporate. Divide batter evenly among prepared muffin tins.

4.   Combine topping ingredients in a bowl and toss with a fork. Sprinkle topping evenly on each muffin and drizzle with Carob Extract™.

5.   Bake 20 to 25 minutes, or until a cake tester inserted into muffin comes out clean.

SERVES 12

1 1/2 cups spelt flour

1/2 cup oat flour

2   tablespoons flaxseeds

1/2 teaspoon sea salt

2 teaspoons baking powder 2 large eggs

2 cups 2 percent cow's milk 2 tablespoons olive oil

2 tablespoons applesauce 1 cup cooked wild rice

1.   Preheat waffle maker.

2.   In a large bowl, whisk dry ingredients together until well combined.

3.   In a separate bowl, whisk wet ingredients. Add wet ingredients to dry, and mix until free of lumps. Fold in cooked rice.

4.   Spoon batter into waffle maker just to the rim, close, and cook according to settings on your waffle maker. Waffles should be firm with a slightly crunchy exterior and soft interior.

5.   Serve warm.

SERVES 4

Blueberry- Macadamia Muffins

1 1/2 cups spelt flour 1 cup oat flour

1/2 teaspoon salt

2 teaspoons baking powder 1 teaspoon baking soda

2   large eggs

1/2 cup agave

1/ teaspoon lemon zest

3   tablespoons light olive oil

1/ cup applesauce

1/ cup plus 2 tablespoons 2 percent cow's milk

1/ cup mashed banana (about 1/ medium banana)

1/ cup chopped macadamia nuts

1   cup organic (fresh or frozen) blueberries

1.   Preheat oven to 350 degrees. Line a 12-cup muffin tin with paper liners and set aside.

2.   In a large bowl, combine dry ingredients. Set aside.

3.   In a separate bowl, whisk wet ingredients to combine. Add the wet ingredients to the dry ingredients, stirring to combine. Fold in macadamia nuts and blueberries. Divide batter evenly among prepared muffin tins and bake for 25 to 28 minutes, or until a cake tester inserted into muffin comes out clean.

4.   Let muffins cool before serving.

SERVES 12

3/4 cup spelt flour

1/4 cup oat flour

2   teaspoons baking powder 1/2 teaspoon fine-grain sea salt 2 large eggs

1 cup nonfat cow's milk 2 tablespoons olive oil

1.   Combine flours, baking powder, and salt.

2.   In a separate bowl, whisk eggs, milk, and olive oil. Add to flour mixture and stir until well combined and free of lumps.

3.   Spray a skillet with nonstick cooking spray and place over medium-low heat. Spoon 1/ cup batter into skillet at a time, and let cook 1 to 2 minutes per side.

4.   Serve warm. (If making a large batch, keep pancakes in the oven at 200 degrees, draped with a slightly damp paper towel.)

SERVES 4

scones:

1/2 cup dried cherries, halved

1   cup spelt flour, plus more for rolling

1/2 cup oat flour

1/4 cup almond flour

2   teaspoons baking powder

1/2 teaspoon sea salt

4 tablespoons butter, chilled 1/4 cup 2 percent cow's milk 1 large egg

1   teaspoon lemon zest

1/3 cup agave

topping:

2   tablespoons agave

2 tablespoons almond flour

1.   Preheat oven to 350 degrees. Line a baking sheet with parchment paper and set aside.

2.   Place dried cherries in a small bowl and cover with steaming-hot water for 10 minutes to rehydrate. Remove, pat dry, and set aside.

3.   In a large mixing bowl, combine flours with baking powder and salt.

4.   Cut butter into small cubes and cut into the flour mixture using a pastry cutter or two butter knives until mixture resembles coarse cornmeal. Toss cherries into dry mixture, making sure they are evenly distributed throughout the flour mixture.

5.   In a separate bowl, whisk milk, egg, lemon zest, and agave until well combined. Fold the milk mixture into the flour mixture until well combined.

Dough will be thick and slightly sticky. If necessary, use extra flour to gather the dough into a ball. Gently place on a floured surface and use your hands to pat the dough into a 1-inch-thick rectangle. Using a sharp knife, cut the dough horizontally once and then into thirds vertically, to make 6 squares. Cut each square again at an angle, to make 12 triangles. Gently place each scone on prepared baking sheet. Brush the tops evenly with agave and almond flour.

6.   Bake 20 to 22 minutes or until scones are firm and lightly browned on the bottom.

7.   Serve warm or let cool completely and store in a cool, dry place overnight. (Scones can be frozen and reheated for up to a month. Reheat at 200 degrees for 10 minutes.)

SERVES 12

tip: Keeping all ingredients—and your mixing bowls—cold creates a flaky texture in your scones.

1/ fresh pear

3/ cup spelt flour

1/ cup oatmeal flour

1   tablespoon finely chopped fresh rosemary

1/ teaspoon sea salt

2   teaspoons baking powder 2 large eggs

1/ cup agave

1/ cup extra virgin olive oil

1/ cup chopped walnuts

1.   Preheat oven to 350 degrees. Grease 81/ " x 41/ " loaf pan with oil from a refillable oil mister and set aside.

2.   Peel and dice a ripe pear into small pieces and set out on a paper towel to drain excess water.

3.   In a large bowl, whisk flours, rosemary, salt, and baking powder to combine.

4.   In a separate bowl, whisk eggs, agave, and olive oil until well combined. Add the wet ingredients to the flour mixture and stir to combine. Fold in chopped walnuts and drained pears.

5.   Spoon batter into prepared loaf pan. Bake 30 to 35 minutes, or until cake tester comes out clean.

SERVES 10

tip: Refillable spray cans are widely available, so fill with allowable oil and use as nonstick spray.

Chapter 3: Lunch recipes

lunch recipe provides a balance between vegetables and varying types of proteins while staying lighter on the complex carbohydrates. Recipes that

are more dominantly vegetable or protein include suggestions for a tasty complement of the other.

2 slices brown rice bread

1/ teaspoon olive oil Large-grain sea salt, to taste 2 tablespoons Navy Bean Hummus*

1 (1/ -inch-thick) slice brick feta cheese 3 thin-sliced rounds green bell pepper 2 leaves Boston Bibb lettuce

1.   Toast bread lightly until honey brown, and drizzle one side of each slice with olive oil and a scant sprinkling of sea salt.

2.   Smear hummus on the olive oil side of one piece of toast, and top with feta, sliced bell peppers, and lettuce leaves. Place the second piece of toast oil side down, and slice in half.

3.   Serve immediately.

SERVES 2

meatballs:

1 pound lean, ground, organic lamb

1/ cup grated onion 1/ cup finely chopped fresh mint 1/ teaspoon sea salt 1 teaspoon curry powder

1 large egg

5 tablespoons bread crumbs*

pimiento sauce:

2 teaspoons olive oil

1/ cup onions, chopped 1 clove garlic, minced 1 (4.2-oz.) jar pimientos, drained and chopped 1/ cup Vegetable Stock*

Sea salt, to taste 1 teaspoon agave

1/ cup fresh basil, chopped 4 brown rice or millet buns

1/ cup mozzarella 1. Preheat oven to 400 degrees. Line a baking sheet with parchment paper and set aside.

2.   Combine all meatball ingredients in a large bowl and gently combine with your hands. Try not to overwork the meat because it will get too tough.

3.   Roll meatballs into golf ball–size pieces and place 2 inches apart on prepared baking sheet. Bake for 20 minutes or until golden brown and cooked through.

4.   While meatballs cook, prepare pimiento sauce. In a high-sided skillet, heat olive oil over medium heat. Sauté onion and garlic, 5 to 6 minutes. Add chopped pimientos, agave, and stock and bring to a boil. Reduce to a gentle bubble, and let cook 10 to 15 minutes. Add salt, to taste.

5.   When meatballs are done cooking, add to sauce and toss to coat. Spoon onto buns and top with cheese and basil.

6.   Serve warm.

SERVES 4

fish:

1 pound haddock

1/4 teaspoon sea salt 1 large egg, slightly beaten

1/2 cup spelt flour 1 teaspoon garlic powder 1 tablespoon olive oil

sauce:

1 (5.5-oz.) container thick low-fat Greek yogurt 1 tablespoon minced onion

Sea salt, to taste

1 tablespoon chopped fresh dill 2 teaspoons lemon zest

4 spelt or brown rice buns

1   cup shredded romaine lettuce

1.   Season haddock with sea salt, and slice into 4 individual fillets. In one large,

flat-bottomed bowl, add beaten egg, and in a second combine flour and garlic powder. Dip each haddock fillet into the egg and then into the flour mixture. Dust off excess flour, and place onto a clean plate.

2.   In a large, high-sided skillet, heat olive oil over medium heat. Add fish fillets, keeping 2 inches of space between each. Cook about 4 minutes per side or until center is flaky and opaque.

3.   Make yogurt sauce by whisking all sauce ingredients in a small bowl.

4.   Toast buns, spoon yogurt sauce on each bun half, and top with romaine and cooked fish.

SERVES 4

tip: Keep an eye on the fish while it cooks to make sure it does not burn. You may need to flip the fish twice to make sure this does not happen. If more oil is needed, add 1 teaspoon at a time.

2   teaspoons olive oil, divided

4 strips (nitrate-and preservative-free) turkey bacon 4 cups spinach

4 teaspoons ghee 4 slices oat bread

1/2 cup shredded mozzarella cheese 1. Preheat oven to 200 degrees.

2.   Heat 1 teaspoon olive oil in a medium skillet over medium heat. Cook bacon for 1 to 2 minutes per side. Drain on paper towel and keep warm in oven until you are ready to add it to the grilled cheese. This will help the bacon crisp up further.

3.   In same skillet, sauté spinach in remaining 1 teaspoon olive oil over medium heat for 1 to 2 minutes, just until leaves are wilted.

4.   Spread ghee evenly on one side of each piece of bread. Place bacon, spinach, and cheese on unbuttered side of bread, and top with a second piece of buttered bread, so that the outer side of each piece is buttered. Cook in skillet over medium heat until lightly browned on each side and cheese has melted.

5.   Slice in half and serve warm.

SERVES 2

salad:

1 head escarole

1/2 cup canned white beans, drained and rinsed 2 cups snap peas 4 cups string beans

dressing:

1 tablespoon fresh mint

1 tablespoon fresh lime juice

1/ teaspoon ground cumin 1 clove garlic, minced

1/ teaspoon honey 1/ cup olive oil Sea salt, to taste

1.   Wash escarole and pat dry. Tear escarole into bite-size pieces and place into a large serving bowl, top with white beans, and set aside.

2.   Bring a large pot of water to boil. Boil snap peas and string beans for 3 minutes, drain, and shock in a large bowl of ice water to stop the cooking process. Lay the peas and beans on a kitchen towel to dry, and add to escarole mixture.

3.   Whisk together all dressing ingredients in a small bowl. Drizzle over salad and serve.

SERVES 4

crust:

1/4 cup shaved hard goat cheese Store-bought spelt crust (with allowable grains)

salad:

1 head broccoli

1   teaspoon olive oil Sea salt, to taste

2   cups watercress

1 cup beets, diced and roasted

1 tablespoon blanched, slivered almonds

dressing:

1 tablespoon fresh lemon juice

1   teaspoon minced onion 1 tablespoon olive oil

2   teaspoons diced fresh oregano

1.   Preheat oven to 375 degrees.

2.   Spread goat cheese evenly on top of pizza crust, and bake 3 to 4 minutes until cheese begins to melt. Remove and let cool.

3.   Increase oven temperature to 400 degrees. Cut broccoli into bite-size florets, place on a baking sheet, and toss with olive oil and sea salt. Bake for 20 minutes. Remove from oven and cool completely.

4.   In a small bowl, whisk together all dressing ingredients. Drizzle over watercress, beets, broccoli, and almonds, and toss to combine.

5.   Top crust with salad mixture and serve cold.

SERVES

Dandelion Greens with Roasted Roots and Horseradish Dressing

greens:

1   raw beet

2   parsnips

1   head cauliflower

2   teaspoons olive oil

2 bunches dandelion greens Sea salt, to taste

dressing:

1/ cup olive oil 1/ cup grated fresh horseradish 1 tablespoon fresh, chopped basil

2 tablespoons fresh lemon juice Sea salt, to taste

1.   Preheat oven to 375 degrees.

2.   Peel beet and parsnips. Dice beet into 1/ -inch cubes, and slice parsnips into 1/ - inch pieces. Remove outer leaves from cauliflower, and cut into bite-size florets. Toss vegetables with olive oil, and season with sea salt. Spread in a single layer on a baking sheet, and bake for 55 to 60 minutes, tossing halfway through. Vegetables should be easily pierced with fork and slightly browned on the edges and bottoms.

3.   To prepare dressing, grate fresh horseradish. In a small bowl, whisk all dressing ingredients to combine.

4.   Toss dandelion greens in a large bowl with horseradish dressing, top with roasted vegetables, and serve.

SERVES 4

salad:

2 cups cubed eggplant 2 teaspoons olive oil Sea salt, to taste

6 cups torn romaine lettuce

1/ cup sliced pepperoncini peppers 1/ cup feta cheese, rumbled dressing:

1   tablespoon fresh oregano

2   tablespoons fresh-squeezed lemon juice 3 tablespoons olive oil

Sea salt, to taste

1.   Preheat oven to 375 degrees. Spray a baking sheet with nonstick cooking spray.

2.   Place eggplant on prepared baking sheet. Drizzle with olive oil and sprinkle with sea salt. Bake for 35 minutes, until eggplant is softened and slightly browned on the bottom. Remove from oven, and let cool.

3.   In the bottom of a large bowl, whisk dressing ingredients together, and set aside.

4.   Wash lettuce, and pat dry. Tear into bite-size pieces, and place in a serving bowl. Add roasted eggplant, peppers, and feta cheese. Drizzle with dressing and toss to combine.

SERVES 4

1 head radicchio

1/ pound salmon, cooked 3 tablespoons chopped chives

1/ teaspoon sea salt 1/ cup cooked peas 1/ cup finely diced apples 1 teaspoon honey

1   teaspoon chopped fresh oregano Juice of 1 lemon

Zest of 1 lime

1/ cup olive oil 1. Peel outer leaves of radicchio, and discard the first couple leaves. Continue peeling inner leaves gently, snapping at the base to maintain the integrity of each leaf. Clean with cold water and let dry on a kitchen towel.

2.   Flake salmon into a bowl, and add chives, salt, peas, and apples.

3.   In a small bowl, whisk together honey, oregano, lemon juice, lime zest, and olive oil. Drizzle over salmon mixture, and toss gently to combine.

4.   Spoon salmon salad into prepared radicchio cups.

SERVES 2

11/2   cups dried navy beans (not canned or precooked) 1 tablespoon olive oil, divided

1/2 cup chopped parsley 2 tablespoons spelt flour 1 cup chopped onion

2   cloves garlic, minced

1/4 teaspoon coriander 1/4 teaspoon cumin 1/4 teaspoon sea salt 1. Soak dry beans overnight in cold water, drain, and rinse.

2.   Boil presoaked beans for 30 minutes, drain, and rinse. Beans should be almost completely cooked, but remain a firm texture. Set beans in a single layer on a paper towel to dry.

3.   Preheat oven to 350 degrees. Brush a baking sheet with 1 to 2 teaspoons olive oil, and set aside.

4.   In a food processor, add beans, parsley, flour, onion, garlic, coriander, cumin, and salt. Pulse until ingredients form a thick paste. Use a tablespoon to scoop

mixture into the palm of your hand and roll into balls and place on prepared baking sheet. Repeat until all of the mixture has been used. Brush remaining olive oil on the tops of falafel balls and bake for 25 minutes.

5.   Increase the oven temperature to 400 degrees, and bake an additional 15 minutes. Falafels will be cooked through, warm and firm through the center.

6.   Serve on top of Roasted-Eggplant Greek Salad.*

SERVES 4

salad:

1   bunch kale

2   teaspoons olive oil

1   large white onion, sliced

1/ cup raisins dressing:

2   tablespoons olive oil 2 limes, juiced

1 clove garlic, minced

1/ teaspoon ground cumin Sea salt, to taste

1.   Wash kale and dry on kitchen towels. Strip kale off the woody stems by holding the stem with one hand, wrapping finger and thumb of the other hand around the stem, and pulling quickly down. Discard stems and tear leaves into bite-size pieces. Place in a large bowl and set aside.

2.   Heat olive oil in a skillet over medium heat. Add onion, and sauté 3 to 4 minutes. Add raisins, and continue cooking for 5 minutes. Remove from heat and toss with raw kale.

3.   In a small bowl, whisk together dressing ingredients. Drizzle over kale salad and toss to coat. Serve with leftover or chilled baked salmon or beans for added protein.

SERVES 4

spring rolls:

3 small, tricolored carrots 1 cup thinly sliced kale

1 orange bell pepper, thinly sliced

1/ cup finely sliced red onion 1/ cup julienned fresh basil 2 teaspoons olive oil Sea salt, to taste

4 rice paper wraps

sweet cherry dip:

1/ cup (no sugar added) cherry jam 1 tablespoon fresh grated ginger 1 tablespoon finely diced onion

1   teaspoon agave

Juice of 1/ lemon Sea salt, to taste

1.   Peel and slice carrots into thin matchsticks.

2.   Toss kale, bell pepper, carrots, onion, and basil together in a bowl with olive oil and sea salt, to taste. Set aside.

3.   Pour hot water halfway up a large, flat-bottomed bowl. One at a time, submerge rice paper wraps in water until they soften and become pliable, about 30 seconds. Rice paper will be delicate, so be gentle. Place rice paper on a placemat or cutting board and spoon about 2 tablespoons vegetable mixture down the center of the rice paper. Roll the sides over the vegetables first and then pull the top over the vegetables and continue to roll up. Slice in half and repeat until remaining rice papers and filling are used.

4.   In a small saucepan, combine all sauce ingredients over low heat. Stir 1 to 2 minutes until warmed through and melted together.

5.   Serve wraps with cherry dip.

SERVES 2

featured ingredient

rice paper wraps

Typically found in Asian markets, rice paper is used to make spring rolls, and thanks to its increased popularity, can now be found at most natural or health food stores. It is made of rice and water, and when dried, resembles stiffened parchment paper that looks pretty inedible. When soaked in warm water, however, rice paper transforms to a pliable, tender state, and can be used as a delicate wrap for fresh delicious flavors that get tucked inside like a burrito. Rice paper comes in packages of 50 to 100 papers and costs close to nothing, so it is a great, low-calorie, low-budget addition to your culinary repertoire.

crust:

2   tablespoons quinoa flour

1/3 cup millet flour 2/3 cup brown rice flour 1/2 teaspoon sea salt 4 tablespoons cold unsalted butter or ghee

5 tablespoons ice-cold water

filling:

2 teaspoons olive oil 4 cups baby spinach

2 cups chopped red kale

1   cup diced yellow pepper

1/ cup diced white onion 1 cup feta cheese 2 large eggs

1/ cup Vegetable Stock*

2   tablespoons fresh thyme Sea salt, to taste

1.   Preheat oven to 375 degrees.

2.   Make crust by tossing flours and salt. Cut cold butter into small pieces and add to flour mixture. Using a crossing motion with two butter knives or a pastry cutter, incorporate butter into the flour until the mixture resembles coarse cornmeal. Add water, 1 tablespoon at a time, until the dough comes together but is not sticky. Gather dough in your hands and knead until it becomes smooth and pliable. Small pieces of butter should still be visible. Place in a bowl and cover dough with plastic wrap. Refrigerate 1 hour.

3.   Roll dough on a flat, floured surface until about 12 inches in diameter and approximately 1/-inch thick. Place into a 9-inch pie plate and gently press the dough into the pan, pinching edges between two fingers to create crimped edges.

4.   Par-bake crust for 15 minutes. Par-baking means partially baking a crust to firm the crust before adding filling.

5.   Prepare filling while crust bakes. Heat olive oil in large skillet over medium heat. Sauté spinach, kale, pepper, and onion for about 4 minutes, just until vegetables are tender. Transfer vegetables to a large bowl, toss with feta, and set aside to cool.

6.   In a separate bowl, whisk eggs, stock, thyme, and sea salt, to taste. Pour over cooled vegetables, and mix to combine.

7.   Pour filling into par-baked crust, and bake 30 minutes or until filling is firm.

8.   Serve warm or cold (if serving cold, let cool and then place in refrigerator until ready to eat).

SERVES 6

2 teaspoons olive oil 1 cup diced onion

1   celery root (celeriac), peeled and diced 2 cups diced orange bell pepper

2   cans organic kidney beans, drained and rinsed 11/2 cups Vegetable Stock*

1 clove garlic

1 sprig sage

4 sprigs thyme

1 teaspoon sea salt 2 cups snow peas

1.   In a large Dutch oven, heat olive oil over medium heat. Add onion and celery

root, sautéing 4 to 5 minutes. Add orange pepper and sauté an additional 2 to 3 minutes. Vegetables should be tender and aromatic. Add remaining ingredients and bring to a gentle boil.

2.   Reduce heat, cover, and simmer 25 minutes, until vegetables are soft and warmed through. Add snow peas and cook a final 5 minutes.

3.   Remove sage and thyme sprigs, then serve warm.

SERVES 4

Chapter 4: Dinner recipes

he bulk of the recipes in this book are in this section. Here you will find a variety of dishes from pastas to seafood, all-in-one dishes, and so on. Most of the recipes are simple to make, but others take a bit more time to prepare. Hopefully these dishes inspire you to take some time to enjoy delicious, wholesome food for yourself and your family.

1   large head broccoli

2   large red bell peppers 1 tablespoon olive oil

5 sprigs thyme, divided Sea salt, to taste

1   tablespoon plus 2 teaspoons ghee, divided

1/2 cup bread crumbs*

2   tablespoons white or brown rice flour 2 cups Vegetable Stock*

1 cup 2 percent cow's milk 2 sprigs sage, chopped

1 pound brown rice or quinoa elbow pasta 1 cup shredded mozzarella cheese

1/2 cup cubed fresh mozzarella cheese

1.   Preheat oven to 375 degrees.

2.   Cut broccoli and bell peppers into bite-size pieces. Place in a single layer on a baking sheet, drizzle with olive oil, and salt. Strip leaves from thyme sprigs and sprinkle over the vegetables. Bake for 30 minutes, until the vegetables are tender and slightly browned. Set aside.

3.   Melt 2 teaspoons ghee, toss with bread crumbs and a pinch of sea salt, and set aside.

4.   Make a roux by melting remaining 1 tablespoon of ghee in a saucepan over

medium-low heat and whisking in rice flour until well combined into a paste. Gradually add stock and milk to flour mixture, whisking after each addition until smooth and free of lumps. Add sage and increase heat to medium. Bring to a boil, whisking constantly. Reduce heat to a simmer and cook until the roux thickens, about 10 minutes. Add salt, to taste.

5.   Cook pasta according to package instructions (if using brown rice pasta, cook 3 to 4 minutes short of recommended cooking time). Drain pasta and pour into casserole dish. Toss with roasted vegetables. Cover pasta with sauce and shredded mozzarella cheese, gently tossing with pasta to incorporate throughout the dish. Top with reserved bread crumbs and fresh mozzarella.

6.   Bake 20 to 25 minutes, until hot and bubbling, and the bread crumbs are golden brown and toasted.

SERVES 6

1 pound spelt or brown rice spaghetti 2 teaspoons olive oil

1/2 cup diced onions

4 slices turkey bacon 2 cups asparagus

3 cups sliced red kale 2 large eggs

2 egg yolks

1/4 cup 2 percent cow's milk Sea salt, to taste

1/ cup ricotta cheese

1.   Bring a large pot of salted water to a boil. Cook spaghetti according to package directions (if using brown rice spaghetti, cook 4 minutes short of package cooking time). Drain, reserving 1/ cup pasta cooking water, and set aside.

2.   Heat olive oil in a large, high-sided skillet over medium heat. Sauté onions for 4 to 5 minutes. Chop turkey bacon into about 1/ -inch pieces and add to the pan, sautéing until browned, about 5 to 6 minutes. Remove turkey bacon and onions and set aside.

3.   Slice asparagus spears in quarters and add to skillet with kale. Sauté until vegetables are tender, about 3 to 4 minutes. Add bacon and onion back to the skillet and reduce heat to low.

4.   In a bowl, whisk together eggs, yolks, milk, and salt, to taste. Slowly pour reserved pasta cooking water into the egg mixture to temper the eggs. Remove the skillet from the heat, add cooked pasta to vegetables, and pour egg mixture over top. The heat from the pasta will gently cook the eggs and create a sauce. Stir in cheese and season with salt.

5.   Serve immediately.

SERVES 6

1   bunch asparagus 1 bunch beet greens

2   large bunches kale, divided

1/2 cup plus 3 teaspoons olive oil Sea salt, to taste

1   pound brown rice pasta Juice of 1 lemon

1/ cup walnuts

2   cloves garlic, minced

1/ teaspoon cracked red pepper, plus extra for serving 3 slices nitrate- /preservative-free turkey bacon

1/ cup Gouda cheese, grated

2 cups cooked peas Zest of 1 lemon

1.   Preheat oven to 375 degrees.

2.   Tear beet greens into bite-size pieces and place them in a large bowl. Snap asparagus spears close to the bottom, and discard the woody stems. Cut into bite- size pieces and toss with beet greens. Tear 11/ bunches kale into large bite-size pieces and add to bowl. Toss vegetables with 2 teaspoons olive oil and a pinch of salt.

3.   Place on a baking sheet, and bake for 12 minutes or until vegetables are tender and kale has slightly crispy edges. Set aside. Reduce oven temperature to 200 degrees.

4.   Bring a large pot of water to boil. Cook pasta 4 minutes short of recommended cooking time.

5.   While pasta is cooking, prepare pesto. Tear remaining kale into bite-size pieces; you'll have about 21/ cups. Combine with 1/ cup olive oil, lemon juice, walnuts, garlic, salt, and pepper in a food processor, and pulse until smooth. Spoon into a bowl and set aside.

6.   Cook bacon in a skillet with remaining 1 teaspoon olive oil until crispy, about 2 minutes per side. Wrap in a damp paper towel and keep warm in the oven until ready to serve, to make bacon extra crispy.

7.   Drain pasta and place in a large pasta bowl. Toss immediately with pesto, cheese, peas, and roasted vegetables. Sprinkle with cracked red pepper and lemon zest. Crumble bacon and sprinkle on top. Serve warm.

SERVES 6

gnocchi:

2 cups sweet potato, boiled

3/4 cup brown rice flour

1/4 cup millet flour 1 teaspoon sea salt 1 large egg, beaten

1/4 teaspoon fresh ground nutmeg

sauce:

1   tablespoon olive oil 1 teaspoon ghee

1/4 cup finely diced shallots

1/2 cup Vegetable Stock* 1 tablespoon lemon juice 1/4 cup dried cranberries

1/2 cup torn fresh basil

1.   Mash boiled sweet potatoes with a fork or potato masher until smooth and creamy.

2.   In a large bowl, combine smashed sweet potatoes with remaining gnocchi ingredients. Use your hands to lightly form into a dough ball. If the dough is too sticky, sprinkle more brown rice flour over the dough. Grab a handful of dough at a time and roll on a floured surface into long, 3/4-inch-thick cylinders. Repeat with remaining dough.

3.   Use a sharp knife to slice the cylinders into 1-inch pieces. Roll each piece gently over the back of a fork, to make indentations in the gnocchi.

4.   Bring a large pot of salted water to a gentle boil. Drop gnocchi into the water in batches, being careful to not crowd the pot. The gnocchi will float to the top when they are finished cooking, about 2 to 3 minutes. Remove with a slotted spoon and transfer to a baking sheet until all gnocchi has been cooked.

5.   Heat olive oil and ghee in a large skillet over medium heat. Sauté shallots for 2 to 3 minutes. Add stock, lemon juice, and cranberries.

6.   Toss gnocchi with sauce just to coat, garnish with basil, and serve warm.

SERVES 4

infused oil:

Zest of 1/2 lemon

1/3 cup olive oil

1/8 teaspoon mustard powder

1/2 teaspoon cumin seeds 2 cloves garlic, smashed

pesto:

1/4 cup plus 2 tablespoons toasted almonds, divided 2 tablespoons olive oil

1/4 cup chopped fresh sage

1/4 cup grated hard goat cheese 1 cup chopped spinach

2 tablespoons lemon juice 1 teaspoon lemon zest

1/2 teaspoon sea salt 1 tablespoon water

3/4 pound spinach, brown-rice, or spelt spaghetti 2 heads radicchio

1/2 cup kefir cheese, cut into 1-inch dice

1. In a small skillet, combine all infused oil ingredients. Cook over low heat for 15 minutes. Remove from heat and set aside.

2. In a food processor or mini chopper, combine 1/4 cup almonds, olive oil, sage, cheese, spinach, lemon juice, lemon zest, sea salt, and water. Pulse until mixture is pureed and resembles a thick sauce.

3. Cook pasta according to package instructions. If using brown rice pasta, cook 4 minutes short of package instructions.

4.   While the pasta cooks, heat grill pan over medium heat and brush with infused oil. Peel outer layers of radicchio and discard. Cut peeled radicchio in quarters. Brush each quarter with infused olive oil, and grill about 1 minute per side or until radicchio begins to become tender and slightly wilted.

5.   Drain pasta, and toss with pesto and kefir in a large serving bowl. Top with grilled radicchio and reserved toasted almonds.

6.   Serve immediately.

SERVES 2

tip: Store infused oil in a sealed, glass container in a cool, dry place for up to 1 week. Great on salads or drizzled over toast.

lasagna:

5   medium zucchini

6   portabella mushrooms

2 tablespoons plus 2 teaspoons olive oil 11/2   teaspoons sea salt, divided

1 cup finely diced onion

4 cups packed baby spinach

2 cups part-skim ricotta cheese 1/2 cup finely chopped walnuts 1 large egg

Dash of cloves

1   cup shredded mozzarella cheese

pesto:

2   cups packed baby spinach 2 cups packed basil

1/2 teaspoon sea salt 2 cloves garlic

1/4 cup lemon juice

1/4 cup olive oil

1/4 cup walnuts

2 tablespoons water

1.   Preheat oven to 375 degrees.

2.   Trim ends off zucchini and slice in 4 long pieces, about 1/4-inch thick.

3.   Line zucchini and portabella mushrooms in a single layer on baking sheets. Drizzle evenly with 2 tablespoons olive oil and 1 teaspoon sea salt. Roast on top rack of oven for 20 minutes.

4.   Heat remaining 2 teaspoons oil in a large skillet over medium heat. Sauté

onion for 8 to 10 minutes, until tender and translucent. Add spinach and sauté 1 minute, just until spinach wilts. Remove from heat.

5.   In a large bowl, stir together ricotta cheese, walnuts, egg, cloves, and reserved spinach mixture. Set aside.

6.   Remove vegetables from the oven, and let cool while you make the pesto. Reduce oven temperature to 350 degrees.

7.   Place all pesto ingredients in a blender and pulse until smooth.

8.   Assemble lasagna by layering a thin layer of pesto in the bottom of a 9" x 11" baking dish, topped with a layer of roasted zucchini, a layer of ricotta mixture, 1/ cup mozzarella cheese, pesto, mushrooms, ricotta, pesto, remaining zucchini, remaining ricotta, remaining pesto, and remaining mozzarella cheese.

9.   Bake for 25 minutes until cheese is melted and slightly browned on the top. Serve warm.

SERVES 6

2 cups Vegetable Stock* 2 cups water

1   lemon, sliced

11/ pounds salmon 1 pound spelt pasta

Spicy mustard, for serving (optional)

sauce:

2   cups spinach

1 cup basil

1   clove garlic, minced 1 cup northern beans

2   teaspoons lemon zest

1/ cup Vegetable Stock*

1 teaspoon granulated mustard

1.   Fill a high-sided skillet with stock, water, and lemon slices. Bring to a simmer and add salmon. Cover and cook 12 to 15 minutes.

2.   In the meantime, cook pasta according to package instructions.

3.   While pasta and salmon cook, make sauce by pureeing sauce ingredients in a food processor or blender.

4.   Drain pasta and toss with all but 1/ cup of the basil sauce. Top with salmon and drizzle with remaining sauce and spicy mustard, if desired.

5.   Serve immediately.

SERVES 4

1 pound wild-caught salmon fillets 2 teaspoons olive oil, divided

1/2 teaspoon sea salt Zest of 1 lemon

1   tablespoon lemon juice

2   tablespoons fresh grated ginger 1 teaspoon honey

1.   Preheat oven to 400 degrees.

2.   Rub salmon with 1 teaspoon olive oil and season with sea salt.

3.   In a small bowl, mix lemon zest, lemon juice, remaining 1 teaspoon olive oil, ginger, and honey until combined. Brush evenly over the top of salmon.

4.   Bake for 10 to 12 minutes.

5.   Serve with Grilled Garlic-Ginger Bok Choy NS (page 127).

SERVES 2

1 pound cooked wild-caught salmon

1 cup cooked cannellini beans, drained and rinsed 1 teaspoon chopped scallions

1 teaspoon fresh rosemary 1 teaspoon fresh thyme Sea salt, to taste

1   large egg, slightly beaten

1/2 cup bread crumbs* 2 teaspoons olive oil

sauce:

2   tablespoons walnuts 2 tablespoons olive oil 2 tablespoons hot water 1/4 cup cilantro

Sea salt and pepper, to taste

1.   Flake cooked salmon into a bowl, and carefully remove any bones. Add beans, scallions, rosemary, thyme, and sea salt. Gently stir in egg and bread crumbs.

2.   Heat olive oil in skillet over medium heat. Form salmon mixture into patties, until all the mixture is used. Cook 3 to 4 minutes, flip, and cook an additional 3 to 4 minutes on the opposite side.

3.   In a food processor, pulse walnuts until they form a paste. With the processor running, add olive oil and water. Once creamy, add cilantro, salt, and pepper.

4.   Serve salmon cakes warm, drizzled with cilantro-cream sauce.

SERVES 4

1   pound mahimahi

1/8 teaspoon ground coriander 1 teaspoon lemon zest

1/4 teaspoon sea salt

fennel salad:

2   teaspoons chopped fresh parsley 2 teaspoons olive oil

Sea salt, to taste

1   teaspoon lemon zest

2   teaspoons lemon juice

2 cups thinly sliced fennel 1 cup thinly sliced Granny Smith apples

1.   Preheat oven to 350 degrees.

2.   Season mahimahi with coriander, lemon zest, and 1/ teaspoon sea salt. Bake for 12 to 15 minutes or until fish is flaky and white.

3.   While the seafood bakes, whisk parsley, olive oil, sea salt, to taste, lemon zest, and juice in the bottom of a bowl. Add fennel and apple, and toss to combine.

4.   Plate fish, top with fennel salad, and serve immediately.

SERVES 2

1 pound snapper (4 fillets)

1/ teaspoon sea salt

1/ teaspoon chili powder 2 cloves garlic, minced 1 tablespoon olive oil

1 cup thinly sliced peaches 1 cup thinly sliced red onion

1/ cup sliced orange bell peppers

1. Preheat oven to 350 degrees.

2. Cut 4 12-inch x 12-inch pieces of parchment paper. Place snapper in the center of each piece of parchment paper, season with salt, chili powder, garlic, and olive oil. Top with peaches, onions, and bell peppers.

3. Lift side of parchment paper up, fold the edges together, and crease. Starting at the edges, crimp and pinch parchment to seal around the fish.

4. Bake 15 minutes or until fish is flaky and opaque. Serve warm.

SERVES 4

1   pound wild-caught halibut steak 1 teaspoon olive oil

1/ teaspoon sea salt

1/ cup fig jam

2   tablespoons chopped fresh basil 2 teaspoons lemon zest

1 teaspoon lemon juice

1. Preheat oven to 400 degrees.

2. Slice halibut into 2 fillets. Drizzle with olive oil and sea salt.

3. In a small bowl, whisk together remaining ingredients. Spread evenly over top of halibut and place in a baking dish.

4. Bake for 30 minutes or until center is flaky and opaque.

SERVES 2

1–2 dried ancho chili peppers

1/ cup wakame (optional) 2 teaspoons olive oil

1 cup diced onions 1 bulb fennel, diced

1   red bell pepper, diced 1 jalapeno, finely diced 1/ teaspoon turmeric

1/ teaspoon fennel seeds Sea salt, to taste

2   (61/-oz.) cans pimiento 2 bay leaves

2   cups Vegetable Stock* 2 cups water

3/ pound cod

1/ pound wild-caught salmon

1.   Place dried ancho chilies in hot water for 10 to 12 minutes. If using wakame, place in cold water for 10 minutes.

2.   In a stockpot, heat olive oil over medium heat. Sauté onion and fennel in olive oil for 4 to 5 minutes. Add red bell pepper and jalapeno, and sauté an additional 3 to 4 minutes. Season with turmeric, fennel seeds, and sea salt, to taste.

3.   Drain chilies, discard stems and seeds, and set aside.

4.   Drain and rinse wakame, if using, and immediately add to stockpot.

5.   Drain pimientos and pat dry. Puree in a food processor with rehydrated chilies until very smooth. (Use less ancho chilies if you wish to reduce the spice.) Add pimiento mixture and bay leaves to sautéed vegetables with stock and water. Simmer 30 minutes.

6.   While the stew simmers, dice cod and salmon into bite-size pieces. After the stew cooks for 30 minutes, add the seafood and let cook an additional 10 minutes, or until seafood is cooked through.

7.   Serve warm.

SERVES 4

3   teaspoons olive oil, divided 2 cups chopped yellow onion 1 cup diced carrots

2 cups diced red bell pepper 1 jalapeno, diced

2 teaspoons garlic, minced

11/2   cups long-grain brown rice 15 threads saffron

1   teaspoon sea salt, plus more, to taste 1 teaspoon paprika

1/8 teaspoon cayenne pepper

1/4 cup chopped parsley

2   cups Vegetable Stock* 1 cup water

1   bay leaf

2   teaspoons fresh oregano

3/ pound halibut fillets

3/ pound mahimahi fillets 1 teaspoon dried oregano

1.   Preheat oven to 350 degrees.

2.   In a large Dutch oven or paella pan, heat 1 teaspoon olive oil over medium heat. Sauté onion, carrots, bell peppers, jalapeno, and garlic for 6 to 7 minutes, stirring frequently. Vegetables should become tender, but not brown. Remove vegetables from pan and set aside.

3.   Add remaining olive oil to the same pan, and toast rice for 2 minutes, stirring constantly. After 2 minutes, the rice will start to smell slightly nutty and darken in color. Add saffron, sea salt, paprika, and cayenne pepper.

4.   Return vegetables to the Dutch oven with the rice and stir to combine. Add parsley, stock, water, bay leaf, and oregano. Bring to a simmer and cover. Place in preheated oven for 40 minutes.

5.   While the paella cooks, dice seafood into 1-inch pieces, and toss with dried oregano and sea salt, to taste.

6.   After 40 minutes, remove paella from oven, and add seafood pieces. Re-cover and bake an additional 12 minutes, until rice absorbs all the liquid.

7.   Seafood should be flaky and opaque when fully cooked, and rice will be fluffy and tender.

8.   Serve warm.

SERVES 6

4 teaspoons olive oil, divided, plus more for greasing 2 cloves garlic

1/ cup parsley

1   teaspoon lemon zest 1 teaspoon sea salt

11/ pounds halibut, skin on 1 red onion

2   white onions, chopped

3   large carrots, peeled and chopped 2 cups green cabbage, shredded

1/ cup fish stock or Vegetable Stock*

1.   Preheat oven to 350 degrees. Drizzle a 9" x 11" baking dish with olive oil to create a nonstick surface for the halibut, and set aside.

2.   In a mini chopper or food processor, puree garlic with parsley, lemon zest, sea salt, and 2 teaspoons olive oil. Set aside.

3.   Season halibut with sea salt. In a large skillet, heat 1 teaspoon olive oil over medium-high heat. Sear halibut, flesh side down for 2 minutes, just to create a crispy crust on the fish. Remove, place skin-side down in prepared baking dish, and top with parsley puree. Set aside.

4.   To the same skillet, add onions, carrots, and cabbage. Sauté over medium heat in the remaining olive oil for about 5 minutes to soften the vegetables slightly. Add salt, to taste. Add stock and stir to deglaze bottom of pan. Pour the carrot mixture around the halibut in the baking dish. Cover and bake 12 minutes (cooking time will vary based on the thickness of the fish). Remove cover and continue to bake for an additional 5 minutes. Halibut should be flaky and bright white all the way through.

5.   Remove dish from the oven. If sauce is runny, remove fish and vegetables and set aside, place the baking dish over medium heat on the stovetop, and stir the liquid to thicken the sauce.

6.   Serve warm.

SERVES 4

fish:

1/4 teaspoon chili powder

1/8 teaspoon cumin

1/2 teaspoon salt

1/4 teaspoon paprika

1 tablespoon plus 1 teaspoon olive oil, divided 1 pound mahimahi

mango salad:

1 finely sliced fennel bulb

1	tablespoon chopped fresh mint

1/2 teaspoon lime zest 1 lime

2	teaspoons olive oil

1/2 cup diced mango

1/2 cup cooked northern beans, drained and rinsed

1/4 teaspoon sea salt

taco crêpes:

2 eggs

1/2 teaspoon sea salt

2/3 cup brown rice flour

1/3 cup spelt flour

1 tablespoon olive oil

11/2 cups 2 percent cow's milk

1.	In a small bowl, combine chili powder, cumin, salt, paprika, and 1 tablespoon olive oil. Slice fish into 1-inch cubes, place in a large bowl, and drizzle spice mixture over fish. Marinate in the refrigerator for at least 20 minutes.

2.	While the fish marinates, make the mango salad. Peel rind and pith off the lime. Carefully cut lime sections away from membrane with a paring knife. Place lime sections and all remaining salad ingredients in a large bowl, toss to combine, and set aside. Allowing the salad to sit while preparing the rest of the dish enables the flavors to combine and textures to soften slightly.

3. To prepare taco crêpes, whisk all crêpe ingredients together in a large bowl. Heat a large skillet or crêpe pan over medium to medium-high heat. (If not using a nonstick pan, use a nonstick cooking spray.) Once hot, spoon 1/4 cup of the crêpe batter onto the skillet and quickly turn the skillet to spread batter in a very thin layer. Let cook about 1 minute, or until the edges start to pull away from the skillet and tiny bubbles appear in the center of the crêpe. Using a large, flat

spatula or carefully lifting edges with your hands, flip the crêpe, and cook 1 additional minute on the other side. Repeat with remaining batter. Stack crêpe on a plate and keep warm until serving.

4. Brush a heated grill pan with remaining 1 teaspoon olive oil, and grill fish 2 to 3 minutes per side, until fish is flaky and opaque.

5. To assemble tacos, place taco crêpe on a plate and top with fish and mango salad.

6. Serve immediately.

SERVES 4

1 tablespoon fresh oregano 2 tablespoons fresh thyme 2 tablespoons fresh basil

1 tablespoon plus 1 teaspoon butter, divided 1 tablespoon olive oil, divided

1/2 cup shallots, minced

3/4 cup chopped figs 2 cups chopped kale

1/4 cup Parmesan cheese (NS omit Parmesan cheese) 1 large, boneless turkey breast

1 tablespoon brown rice flour

1   cup Turkey* or Vegetable Stock*

1.   Preheat oven to 350 degrees.

2.   Finely chop fresh herbs and place in a small bowl. Set aside.

3.   Heat butter and 2 teaspoons olive oil in a large skillet over medium heat. Sauté shallots for 2 to 3 minutes. Add figs and kale, and sauté an additional 4 to 5 minutes. Remove from heat, mix in Parmesan cheese, and set aside.

4.   Slice turkey breast in half to create two pieces. Butterfly turkey breasts by placing on a cutting board and carefully slicing horizontally through the meat, leaving a 1-inch border. This opens the breast so that stuffing it is made simple. Divide kale stuffing evenly between turkey breasts. Gently pull turkey back together and fasten with toothpicks. Sprinkle both sides of stuffed turkey breasts with reserved herb mixture.

5.   Heat oven-safe skillet over medium heat, and add remaining olive oil. Sear stuffed turkey breasts, 3 to 4 minutes per side. Transfer skillet to oven and bake for 8 to 10 minutes or until juices run clear and the internal temperature of the turkey reaches 165 degrees.

6.   Remove turkey from pan and set on a cutting board to rest. Place baking dish over medium heat and add flour and remaining 1 tablespoon butter, whisking

into a paste. Slowly add stock, whisking constantly to form a gravy. Bring to a simmer and cook 2 to 3 minutes, until the gravy coats the back of a spoon.

7.   Slice turkey breasts and drizzle with gravy. Serve warm.

SERVES 4

2   teaspoons ghee

1 bunch broccolini, roughly chopped

1/2 red onion, diced Sea salt, to taste

1/4 cup walnuts

1/3 cup feta cheese, crumbled

1 cup Vegetable Stock*, divided 1 pound turkey tenderloin

1 tablespoon olive oil

1 tablespoon brown rice flour 1 tablespoon oregano

1   tablespoon lemon juice

1.   Preheat oven to 350 degrees.

2.   Heat ghee in a large skillet over medium heat. Sauté broccolini and onion until slightly tender, about 2 to 3 minutes. Season with salt, to taste.

3.   Transfer broccolini mixture to a food processor. Add walnuts, cheese, and 1/4 cup Vegetable Stock, and pulse to combine. Filling should be thick and pasty but not too dry, similar in consistency to cookie dough. If mixture looks dry, add additional stock, 1 tablespoon at a time.

4.   Butterfly the turkey tenderloin by positioning the tenderloin with the tip facing you and the thickest part of the meat facing your slicing hand. Put your hand on top of the tenderloin and insert the knife into the thickest part of the meat, carefully cutting across the tenderloin almost until you reach the opposite side. This will create a pocket for the filling.

5.   Spoon broccolini stuffing into tenderloin and secure closed with toothpicks or cooking twine. Season tenderloin with salt.

6.   Heat olive oil in an oven-safe skillet over medium-high heat. Sear tenderloin, about 2 minutes per side. Cover and place in oven for 20 to 25 minutes. Turkey is cooked when juices run clear and the internal temperature reaches 165 degrees.

7.   Remove turkey from skillet and set aside to rest. Return skillet to stovetop and place over medium heat. Add flour and gradually whisk in remaining stock, oregano, and lemon juice. Bring to a bubble and cook until thickened, about 5 minutes. Season gravy with sea salt if needed, and serve over turkey.

SERVES 4

Crispy- Coated Turkey Tenders with Apricot Dipping Sauce

tenders:

2   rice cakes

2 tablespoons Parmesan cheese (NS omit Parmesan cheese) 1 teaspoon sweet paprika

1/ teaspoon sea salt 1 egg

2 teaspoons 2 percent cow's milk

4 turkey tenderloins 1 tablespoon olive oil

dipping sauce:

2 teaspoons dry mustard

2   tablespoons (no sugar added) apricot spread 1 teaspoon lemon juice

1.   Grind rice cakes in a food processor or mini chopper until they are small crumbs. Pour in a shallow bowl and add cheese, paprika, and salt. Toss to combine.

2. In another shallow bowl, whisk together egg and milk. Dip tenderloins in egg mixture and then into rice cake mixture, turning to coat each side.

3. Preheat oven to 375 degrees. Grease a baking sheet with nonstick cooking spray and set aside.

4. Heat oil in a large, oven-safe skillet over medium heat. Brown tenderloins, about 5 minutes per side. Place onto prepared baking sheet, and bake until cooked through, about 8 minutes or until the internal temperature reaches 165 degrees.

5. While the turkey cooks, make the dipping sauce by whisking together mustard, apricot spread, and lemon juice.

6. Serve warm.

SERVES 4

tip: If you do not have an oven-safe skillet, simply wrap plastic handle with tinfoil.

3 teaspoons olive oil, divided 1 cup diced carrots

1 cup diced onion

1 cup diced red bell pepper

2 tablespoons plus 1 teaspoon fresh thyme 2 cups carrot juice

1 cup Vegetable Stock*

1/8 teaspoon salt, plus additional, to taste 11/2 pounds turkey tenderloin

1 tablespoon arrowroot starch 2 tablespoons cold water

1/2 cup quinoa

1 cup bread crumbs*

1/4 cup shredded mozzarella cheese

1/ cup Parmesan cheese (NS omit Parmesan cheese or substitute more shredded mozzarella cheese)

1. Heat 2 teaspoons olive oil in a Dutch oven over medium heat. Add carrots and onion, and sauté for 5 minutes. Add 2 tablespoons thyme, carrot juice, stock, and salt. Stir just to combine and add turkey tenderloin. Bring to a boil, reduce heat to a low simmer, cover, and cook for 11/ hours.

2. Preheat oven to 375 degrees.

3. After 11/ hours, remove turkey, place onto a cutting board, and shred into bite- size pieces. Return to the pot and increase heat to medium, letting the carrot juice reduce slightly. In a small bowl, dissolve arrowroot starch in water. Add to shredded turkey mixture and stir to help the liquid thicken. After 10 minutes, add quinoa and cook an additional 12 minutes.

4. Mix bread crumbs with 1 teaspoon olive oil, 1/ teaspoon salt, and remaining 1 teaspoon fresh thyme. Toss with cheese.

5. Spoon turkey mixture into 6 individual (7-oz.) ramekins, top with bread crumbs and cheese mixture, and bake for 8 to 10 minutes or until turkey mixture is bubbling and topping is melted.

SERVES 6

8 green tea bags

1 pound turkey tenderloins 1 lemon, divided

1/ teaspoon sea salt 1 cup fresh parsley

3 tablespoons olive oil 1 clove garlic

1   tablespoon water

1.   In a high-sided skillet, bring 4 cups water to a boil, and steep the tea bags for 3 minutes. Reduce heat to medium, and add turkey. Slice half the lemon and add to the poaching liquid with sea salt. Cover and let cook 18 to 20 minutes or until internal temperature of turkey reaches 165 degrees.

2.   Puree parsley, olive oil, garlic, juice from the remaining half of the lemon, and water in a food processor until very smooth.

3.   Serve turkey warm, topped with parsley oil.

SERVES 4

filling:

2   teaspoons olive oil

1 cup frozen pearl onions, thawed 1 cup diced baby carrots

1   cup frozen sweet peas, thawed 1 cup diced parsnips

2   tablespoons spelt or oat flour

31/4   cups Turkey Stock* or Vegetable Stock* 11/2   pounds roasted turkey breast, shredded

1/4 teaspoon saffron threads

1/2 teaspoon dry mustard

topping:

1   teaspoon olive oil

2   cups bread crumbs*

2 teaspoons ghee, melted Sea salt, to taste

crust:

Spelt or whole-wheat store-bought crust (containing allowable grains)

1.   Preheat oven to 375 degrees.

2.   In a Dutch oven, heat 2 teaspoons olive oil over medium heat. Sauté onions, carrots, peas, and parsnips for 5 minutes until vegetables just begin to soften. Sprinkle flour over vegetables and add stock, stirring to prevent lumps. Add roasted turkey, saffron, and dry mustard, stirring to combine. Cover and let cook 15 minutes, stirring occasionally.

3.   In the meantime, sauté bread crumbs in 1 teaspoon olive oil and ghee for 3 to 4 minutes. Remove and toss bread crumbs with sea salt, to taste.

4.   Uncover turkey filling, spoon into spelt crust, and top with toasted bread crumbs. Place in the oven for 20 minutes. The crust will be browned around the edges and the turkey mixture should be hot and bubbling.

5.   Serve warm.

tip: I use leftover roasted turkey for this recipe, but if you're roasting from scratch, place a bone-in, skin-on turkey breast on a rack in a roasting pan. Top with your favorite fresh, chopped herbs and bake for 11/ to 2 hours, until the internal temperature reaches 165 degrees.

SERVES 8

2 teaspoons olive oil 1 pound turkey breast 2 cups diced onion

2 cups diced parsnips

2 large sprigs fresh rosemary 4 large sprigs fresh thyme

1 cup water

1 cup Vegetable Stock* 4 cups torn red kale

1. ' Preheat slow cooker to medium.

2. Heat olive oil in a large skillet over medium heat, and sear turkey breast on all sides. Remove from heat and set aside.

3. In the same skillet, add onion and parsnips, and sauté 3 to 4 minutes. Remove from skillet and place in bottom of slow cooker with rosemary and thyme. Place turkey breast on top of vegetables and herbs.

4. Add water and stock to skillet used to sear turkey and increase heat to medium-high to deglaze, scraping up all the bits. Pour liquid and bits over turkey in the slow cooker.

5. Cover and cook 1 hour. Add the kale and cook 1 additional hour.

6. Serve warm.

SERVES 4

1 teaspoon ghee

2 cloves garlic, minced

1/ cup diced onion

1 teaspoon ground cumin 1 teaspoon sea salt

2 teaspoons ancho chili powder 1/ cup pureed pimiento peppers 1/ cup Vegetable Stock*

2 teaspoons almond butter

1 ounce 100 percent dark chocolate, shaved 3 turkey drumsticks

1.   Preheat oven to 325 degrees.

2.   In a large skillet over medium heat, heat ghee. Sauté garlic and onion for 4 to 5 minutes, until tender and slightly browned. Add cumin, sea salt, and chili powder, stir, and cook an additional 2 minutes. Add pimiento puree, stock, and almond butter, stir to combine, and cook 3 to 4 minutes.

3.   Remove from heat, stir in chocolate, and transfer mixture to a food processor. Puree until smooth. As an optional step, push mole sauce through a strainer to have a silky smooth sauce. If you do not mind the texture, however, leave it as is.

4.   Set aside 1/ of the sauce for use after cooking. Remove skin from turkey drumsticks, discard, and coat drumsticks with mole sauce. Place in a baking dish, cover, and bake for 1 to 11/ hours. Check internal temperature to make sure it reaches 165 degrees.

5.   Once cooked, remove from oven and serve warm, topped with reserved mole sauce.

SERVES 2

3 teaspoons olive oil, divided

1 (2-inch) piece ginger, peeled and thinly sliced

3/ pound turkey breast, thinly sliced 2 cups snow peas

1 cup sliced bok choy

1/ cup finely sliced orange bell pepper

1/ cup plum jam

1 tablespoon lemon juice 1 tablespoon lemon zest 1 tablespoon agave

1.   In a large wok or sauté pan, heat 2 teaspoons olive oil over medium heat. Add ginger and sauté 1 minute. Add turkey and stir-fry until cooked, about 3 to 4 minutes. Remove from wok and set aside.

2.   Add remaining olive oil, snow peas, bok choy, and peppers. Stir-fry 3 to 4 minutes. Add turkey back to the wok along with remaining ingredients. Toss to coat and cook an additional 2 minutes.

3.   Serve hot.

SERVES 4

1 teaspoon paprika

1/ teaspoon sea salt

1/ teaspoon chili powder 1 teaspoon dried thyme

1 pound organic lamb steak 3 teaspoons olive oil, divided 1 teaspoon ghee

1 cup diced onions

8 ounces cremini mushrooms, diced 2 cups diced maitake mushrooms

1 tablespoon fresh thyme

1.   Combine paprika, sea salt, chili powder, and dried thyme. Dice lamb steak into 2-inch pieces and sprinkle spice mixture evenly over the lamb, rubbing in with your hands to evenly distribute spices.

2.   In a large sauté pan, heat 2 teaspoons olive oil over medium heat. Sear lamb 3 minutes per side so that the sides are crispy brown and the middle is light pink. Remove from pan and set aside.

3.   In the same skillet, add remaining 1 teaspoon olive oil, ghee, and onion. Sauté 3 to 4 minutes, add mushrooms and fresh thyme, and sauté an additional 8 to 10 minutes until the mushrooms are soft and aromatic. Return lamb to the pan with mushrooms, tossing to combine.

4.   Serve immediately.

SERVES 4

1 pound lamb chops Sea salt, to taste

1/2 cup olive oil

3 cloves garlic, chopped

pesto:

1/ cup fresh spinach 1 bunch fresh mint

1   teaspoon minced garlic

1/ cup extra virgin olive oil

1/ teaspoon sea salt Juice of 1 lemon

1/ cup raw walnuts

1.   Season lamb with salt, place in a sealable glass container. Pour olive oil over lamb, and sprinkle with garlic. Refrigerate at least an hour. Remove from fridge and let come to room temperature.

2.   In a food processor, combine all pesto ingredients and pulse until smooth. Spoon into a small bowl and set aside.

3.   Heat a grill pan over medium heat, and brush with olive oil. Grill lamb 6 to 7 minutes on each side for medium doneness.

4.   Top with pesto and serve alongside Forbidden Black Rice Risotto*.

SERVES 4

2   medium eggplants

1 tablespoon plus 1 teaspoon olive oil, divided Sea salt, to taste

1   cup diced onion

1/ cup raisins

2   cloves garlic, minced

1/ teaspoon cumin

1/ teaspoon ground ginger

1   jalapeno, seeded and finely diced 1 pound lean ground lamb

1/ cup ricotta cheese 1 cup bread crumbs*

1.   Preheat oven to 400 degrees.

2.   Slice eggplants lengthwise, and spoon out flesh and seeds to create an eggplant boat. Roughly chop insides and reserve. Set eggplant on a baking sheet, skin side down, and drizzle with 1 tablespoon olive oil and a pinch of sea salt. Bake for 30 minutes, remove from oven, and set aside.

3.   In the meantime, heat remaining 1 teaspoon olive oil in skillet over medium heat. Add onion and raisins, and sauté about 4 minutes, just until raisins are plump and juicy and onions are opaque. Add reserved eggplant and sauté an additional 5 minutes, until eggplant is soft. Remove from pan and set aside.

4.   In a small bowl, combine garlic, cumin, ginger, and jalapeno. Toss ground lamb with spice mixture and add to skillet. Brown lamb for 5 minutes, breaking up large pieces with a wooden spoon. Add onion and eggplant mixture back to the skillet and toss to combine. Remove from heat and stir in ricotta cheese.

5.   Spoon lamb mixture into roasted eggplant boats, sprinkle with bread crumbs, and bake an additional 20 minutes. Eggplant boats will be tender and browned slightly on the bottom, filling will be warmed through, and bread crumbs will be golden brown. Serve warm.

SERVES 4

2   teaspoons minced garlic 2 teaspoons minced ginger 1/4 teaspoon ground cumin 1/2 teaspoon turmeric

8 ounces lamb fillet

2 teaspoons olive oil, divided 10 cippolini onions, peeled

1 cup chopped carrots 1 cup chopped parsnips 1/2 cup Vegetable Stock*

1 tablespoon lemon juice

1.   In a small bowl, combine garlic, ginger, cumin, and turmeric. Rub spices on lamb fillets. Heat tagine over medium high heat, and brush with 1 teaspoon olive

oil. When the tagine is hot, sear lamb in tagine just until browned on both sides. Remove from tagine and set aside.

2.   To the tagine, add remaining 1 teaspoon olive oil, onions, carrots, and parsnips, and let cook 5 to 6 minutes.

3.   Reduce heat to low. Place pieces of lamb on top of vegetables and add stock and lemon juice. Cover tagine and let cook for 11/ hours (no peeking). After 11/ hours, uncover. Most of the liquid should be absorbed, and lamb and vegetables will be tender. Serve warm.

SERVES 4

tip: A tagine is a Moroccan cooking vessel that has a heavy cast-iron or clay base and a domed, pyramid-shaped top, which creates a slow cooking method that adds moisture to each dish. As an alternative, try a cast-iron skillet and cover with tented tinfoil. Just make sure to seal the top of the skillet.

21/2   teaspoons olive oil, divided 3 cloves garlic, divided

Sea salt, to taste

4 cups sweet potato

1 tablespoon chopped fresh sage

1   tablespoon ghee or butter, divided 6 tablespoons 2 percent cow's milk 1 pound ground lamb

2   teaspoons paprika

2 tablespoons flour (brown rice, spelt, or oat) 11/ cups Beef Stock*

2 cups pearl onions 1 cup peas

2 cups finely diced carrots

1   cup shredded low-moisture mozzarella cheese

1.   Preheat oven to 375 degrees.

2.   Drizzle 1/ teaspoon olive oil over two cloves of garlic and season with sea salt. Wrap in tinfoil and roast for 25 minutes.

3.   While the garlic roasts, dice sweet potatoes into 2-inch pieces, and place in a medium pot with just enough water to cover. Bring to a boil and cook about 12 to 15 minutes, just until tender. Using a hand mixer, beat sweet potatoes with roasted garlic, sage, ghee, and milk. Season with sea salt, to taste.

4.   Reduce oven temperature to 350 degrees.

5.   Heat remaining 2 teaspoons olive oil in a large skillet over medium heat. Brown ground lamb for about 5 minutes, breaking up meat using a flat wooden spoon. Once browned, add paprika, and flour, stirring to coat. Add stock. Bring to a simmer, reduce heat, and cook 5 minutes, until sauce thickens.

6.   Add onions, peas, and carrots to the skillet and stir to combine. Pour into a 9" x 11" baking dish, top with sweet potato mixture, spreading evenly with an offset spatula. Sprinkle on cheese and bake for 30 to 35 minutes, until the pie is hot and the cheese is melted and bubbling.

7.   Serve warm.

SERVES 6

tip: As a time saver, frozen pearl onions can be used in this recipe instead of fresh.

Bamboo skewers, for grilling

marinade:

2   tablespoons fresh lemon juice 1 tablespoon agave

3   tablespoons olive oil

1 tablespoon fresh ginger, minced

1/2 teaspoon sweet paprika 1 teaspoon garlic, minced

kabobs:

1 pound organic beef tips

4 cups pineapple pieces

1   red onion, cut into 1/-inch dice

1.   Soak bamboo skewers in water for up to 1 hour before use to prevent burning.

2.   Whisk together marinade ingredients in a bowl and set aside.

3.   Trim any excess fat off beef. Place in a sealable glass dish, and pour 2/ marinade over the beef, tossing to make sure all sides are coated with the marinade. Cover and place in the refrigerator for 3 hours.

4.   Preheat grill or grill pan.

5.   Alternate steak, pineapple, and onion, and repeat twice on each skewer. Brush pineapple and onion with marinade. Grill for 10 to 12 minutes, flipping halfway through cooking and brushing again with any remaining marinade.

6.   Serve warm.

SERVES 4

2   teaspoons olive oil plus 1 teaspoon, divided

1   cup chopped onion 1 cup chopped carrots 1 teaspoon sea salt

1/2 teaspoon paprika

2   teaspoons dried parsley 1 teaspoon garlic powder 12 ounces venison roast 1 cup Beef Stock*

1/ cup red wine

1.   Turn slow cooker to low.

2.   Heat 1 teaspoons olive oil in a large skillet over medium heat, and sauté onion and carrots for 3 to 4 minutes. Remove vegetables from pan and place in slow cooker.

3.   Combine spices in a small bowl, stirring to combine. Sprinkle spices over roast and gently massage into all sides.

4.   Increase skillet heat to medium to medium-high. Add remaining 1 teaspoon olive oil and brown roast on all sides, cooking 1 to 2 minutes per side.

5.   Remove roast from skillet and place in slow cooker. Pour stock and red wine into skillet to deglaze the pan, and use a flat spatula to loosen any bits stuck to bottom of the pan. Pour mixture over roast in slow cooker. Cover and cook on low for 5 hours.

6.   Serve warm with Brown Rice Salad NS (page 146).

SERVES 4

1   cup red quinoa 2 cups water

2   teaspoons ghee

1/ cup diced shiitake mushrooms 1 cup diced maitake mushrooms 11/ cups diced okra

1/ cup finely diced shallots 1/ teaspoon mustard powder 1/ teaspoon dry ginger

2 cloves garlic, minced

2 tablespoons fresh oregano 3/ cup finely diced pineapple 1 cup Vegetable Stock*

5 eggs, divided

1.   Preheat oven to 350 degrees. Grease a 9" x 11" baking dish with nonstick olive oil spray and set aside.

2.   Combine quinoa and water in a saucepan. Bring to a boil, reduce heat, and simmer for 12 minutes. Remove from heat, fluff with a fork, and set aside.

3.   Heat a large skillet over medium heat, and melt ghee. Add mushrooms, okra, and shallots, and sauté 6 to 7 minutes. Remove from heat and set aside.

4.   In a small bowl, whisk together mustard powder, ginger, garlic, oregano, pineapple, stock, and 1 egg. Set aside.

5.   Toss quinoa with mushroom mixture, and place into prepared baking dish. Pour egg mixture evenly over casserole, and use a fork to make sure the liquid reaches all corners of the casserole.

6.   Bake for 35 minutes, until casserole sets and becomes firm.

7.   Just before removing casserole, fry remaining eggs in a skillet coated with nonstick cooking spray. Serve on top of warm casserole.

SERVES 6

1 pound organic, free-range ground lamb

1/2 onion, grated

1 teaspoon minced garlic

1 tablespoon fresh oregano

1/2 teaspoon sea salt

1   teaspoon ghee or butter

2   cups diced cremini mushrooms

1/2 cup crumbled feta cheese

1.   Place ground lamb in a large bowl. Add grated onion, garlic, oregano, and salt. Use your fingers to combine, but try not to overwork the meat or it will become tough. Shape into 6 patties.

2.   Heat a skillet sprayed with olive oil spray over medium heat. Add burgers and cook 3 to 4 minutes per side, until crunchy brown on each side and tender, light pink in the center.

3.   In a small skillet, heat ghee over medium heat. Sauté mushrooms until browned and tender, and season with sea salt, to taste. Top burgers with mushrooms and feta cheese. Serve warm on brown rice, millet, or spelt buns.

SERVES 6

2 teaspoons olive oil 1 cup diced eggplant

2 jalapenos, finely diced

1   cup diced green bell pepper 1 cup diced red bell pepper

2   cups chopped yellow onion 2 cloves garlic, minced

1   pound ground beef 5 cups spinach

1/ cup Vegetable Stock*

2   teaspoons sweet paprika 1 teaspoon cumin

1 can navy beans, drained and rinsed

1.   Heat olive oil in a large pot over medium heat. Add eggplant, jalapenos, bell peppers, onion, and garlic, and sauté 4 to 5 minutes, until vegetables begin to soften and become aromatic. Remove vegetables from the pot and set aside.

2.   Add meat to the same pot and break apart with a flat spoon or spatula. Once the meat is cooked and crumbled, add vegetables back to the pot and reduce heat to low.

3.   Puree spinach in a food processor or blender with stock to create a smooth sauce.

4.   Add pureed spinach and remaining ingredients to chili. Cover and let simmer at least 45 minutes, stirring occasionally to prevent burning.

5.   Serve warm.

SERVES 4

1 tablespoon olive oil 1 cup diced onions

3/ cup diced carrots

1 tablespoon diced serrano chilies 2 zucchini, diced

1/ teaspoon cumin

3 cups navy beans, cooked and drained 5 cups Vegetable Stock*

1/ teaspoon sea salt

1.   Heat olive oil in a large Dutch oven over medium heat. Add onion, carrots, chilies, zucchini, and cumin, and sauté 6 to 7 minutes.

2.   Add beans and Vegetable Stock, season with sea salt, to taste, and let cook a total of 30 to 35 minutes. Stew should be tender and steaming hot.

3.   Serve warm.

SERVES 4

2 cups cooked kidney beans, drained and rinsed, divided 11/2 cups chopped baby spinach

1/4 cup finely diced red bell pepper

1/2 cup shredded carrot

1   tablespoon plus 2 teaspoons olive oil 1 tablespoon fresh thyme

1/2 teaspoon sea salt

2   cloves garlic, minced

1/2 cup bread crumbs* 1 large egg, beaten Olive oil spray

1.   Place 1 cup of beans in a bowl and smash using a fork or potato masher.

2.   In a large bowl, add mashed beans and all remaining ingredients, mixing gently just to combine. The mixture should be moist but easily held together. Form into 6 patties.

3.   Heat a large skillet sprayed with olive oil spray over medium heat. Add the burgers and cook about 4 minutes per side. Serve warm with caramelized onions, toasted brown rice/millet buns, and crunchy lettuce.

SERVES 6

1 large spaghetti squash

1 tablespoon olive oil, divided

1/2 teaspoon sea salt

1/4 cup very finely diced onion 3 ounces goat cheese

1 cup toasted diced walnuts 1 cup finely diced parsley

1.　　Preheat oven to 350 degrees.

2.　　Carefully halve squash from stem to base and scoop out seeds. Brush 2 teaspoons olive oil and sprinkle sea salt over flesh of squash. Roast, cut-side down, on a baking sheet for 35 to 40 minutes. Squash should be browned on the skin and flesh should be easily pierced with a fork. Remove and cool squash for 5 minutes.

3.　　Heat remaining 1 teaspoon olive oil in a small skillet over medium heat. Sauté onion 4 to 5 minutes, or until tender. Remove from heat and add goat cheese, walnuts, and parsley.

4.　　Take a fork and scrape insides of squash from stem to base. Squash will peel

bowl and toss with goat cheese sauce.

5.　　Serve warm.

SERVES 4

1/2 cup brown rice, uncooked 2 cups shredded zucchini

1/2 cup diced onions

1/2 cup diced carrots

1 large egg, lightly beaten 2 cloves garlic, minced

1/2 cup bread crumbs*

3/4 cup canned kidney beans, drained and rinsed 1 teaspoon paprika

1/2 cup navy beans, pureed

1.   Preheat oven to 350 degrees. Spray a 81/2" × 41/2" loaf pan with nonstick cooking spray and set aside.

2.   Combine rice with 1 cup water and cook according to package instructions. Let cool.

3.   Spoon shredded zucchini onto a double layer of paper towels or cheese cloth and squeeze out excess liquid. Add zucchini to a large bowl with onions, carrots, cooked rice, egg, garlic, bread crumbs, kidney beans, and paprika. Toss to evenly distribute ingredients. Add pureed navy beans, stirring again to combine.

4.   Place bean mixture in prepared loaf pan, using an offset spatula to spread evenly, and bake 25 to 30 minutes. The loaf should hold together and be firm but

5.   Serve warm.

SERVES 4

Chapter 5: Soup and sides

any times when preparing dinner, we think about eating a protein, vegetable, and complex carbohydrate, and although having them all

together in one pot like chili or lasagna is ideal, it doesn't always work out that way. Therefore, it is essential to have a collection of quick, delicious side or soup options to pair with your protein choice. A number of vegetable-or complex carbohydrate–based soups and sides to keep on hand can be found in this section.

2–3 teaspoons olive oil 1 cup diced onion

1 teaspoon garlic, minced

1 tablespoon ginger, minced

1/8 teaspoon turmeric

1/4 teaspoon curry powder 1 jalapeno, cut into

1/4-inch rounds

1 green bell pepper, diced into 1/2-inch cubes 2 small turnips, diced

4 cups water

1 stick lemongrass Sea salt, to taste

1/4 cup 2 percent cow's milk 1 tablespoon sour cream

1.   Heat olive oil in a stockpot over medium heat, Sauté onion, garlic, and ginger for 3 to 4 minutes until slightly tender and aromatic. Add turmeric, curry

powder, jalapeno, bell peppers, and turnips. Stir and cook 5 minutes.

2.   Pour water over vegetables. Bruise lemongrass by hitting it with the blunt edge of your knife to release the essential oils and then add lemongrass to the pot. Cover, and simmer for at least 30 minutes. Season with sea salt, to taste.

3.   Whisk together milk and sour cream in a small bowl and set aside.

4.   Remove lemongrass from soup just before serving. Pour cream mixture into soup, and stir to combine.

5.   Serve warm.

SERVES 6

1 teaspoon olive oil 2 teaspoons ghee

1   cup chopped onion 1 clove garlic

2   pounds carrots, peeled and diced

1 (3-inch) piece or about 1/ cup ginger, peeled and grated

1/ teaspoon sea salt

1 tablespoon lemon zest 4 cups water

1.   In a stockpot, heat olive oil and ghee over medium heat. Add onion, garlic, and carrots, sautéing 5 to 6 minutes until vegetables become tender. Add remaining ingredients and bring to a boil, reduce to a simmer, cover, and cook at least 30 minutes, or until carrots are fork-tender but not falling apart.

2.   Puree soup with an immersion blender or standing blender until smooth. If the mixture appears too thick, add water until desired consistency is reached.

3.   Serve warm.

SERVES 6

4 cups diced parsnips

4 cups diced cauliflower 2 cloves garlic, peeled

2 tablespoons olive oil, divided 2 cups finely sliced sweet onion Sea salt, to taste

2 Granny Smith apples, finely diced 11/ cups 2 percent cow's milk

1 cup water

1/ teaspoon nutmeg

1/ cup chopped fresh sage

1.   Preheat oven to 375 degrees.

2.   Place parsnips, cauliflower, and garlic cloves on a sheet pan, and drizzle with 1 tablespoon olive oil and sprinkle with sea salt. Toss to coat.

3.   Roast vegetables in the oven for 30 to 35 minutes, until tender and slightly golden brown around the edges.

4.   About 15 minutes before the vegetables are finished cooking in the oven, heat remaining 1 tablespoon oil in a large stockpot over medium heat, and sauté onions for 8 to 10 minutes. Add apples, and sauté an additional 2 to 3 minutes.

5.   Once the onions are tender and vegetables are done roasting, add roasted vegetables and remaining ingredients to stockpot. Bring the soup to a gentle boil, reduce heat, and simmer for 20 minutes. Blend with an immersion blender or puree in a standing blender until smooth and creamy.

6.   Season with additional sea salt, to taste.

7.   Serve warm.

SERVES 6

5 large white onions 1 tablespoon olive oil

1/2 tablespoon ghee or butter

1/2 cup red wine 4 sprigs thyme

2 sprigs sage

2   bay leaves Sea salt, to taste

3   cups Beef Stock*

4   slices brown rice/millet bread, toasted 1 cup grated Gruyere cheese

1.   Slice onions in half and then slice into thin, half-moon shapes.

2.   In a large-bottomed stockpot, heat olive oil and ghee over medium heat. Add onions and caramelize for 12 minutes. Season with sea salt, reduce heat to medium-low, and cook an additional 20 minutes. Onions will become a rich, caramel color as the natural sugars in the onions release and sweeten them.

3.   Add wine to the onions to deglaze the pan, and cook another 30 seconds. Add thyme, sage, bay leaves, salt, and stock. Bring to a boil, reduce heat, and simmer 30 minutes.

4.   Spoon soup into 4 (7-oz.) high-sided, oven-safe bowls or ramekins. Top each with 1 slice toast then sprinkle with cheese, to create a cheesy bread lid for the soup.

5.   Broil in oven for 2 minutes or until the cheese begins to bubble and brown slightly. Keep a close eye, as the toast and cheese can burn quickly.

6.   Serve warm.

SERVES 4

1   tablespoon olive oil, divided 1 cup diced white onion

2   heads broccoli

1 clove garlic, minced

1 (15-oz.) can northern beans, drained and rinsed 2 cups Vegetable Stock*

4 sprigs fresh thyme Sea salt, to taste Pine nuts, to garnish

1.   Heat 2 teaspoons olive oil in a stockpot over medium heat, add onion, and sauté 5 to 6 minutes.

2.   Trim woody stems off broccoli and discard. Roughly chop the broccoli and remaining stems. Add to the onions along with garlic, beans, stock, and thyme. Bring to a boil, reduce heat, and simmer for 15 minutes. Vegetables should be tender and easily pierced with a fork, but not falling apart.

3.   Puree soup using an immersion blender, or puree in batches in a regular blender, until smooth. Soup should be thick and creamy, but easily run off your spoon. Add water or additional stock if you prefer a thinner consistency. Season with sea salt, to taste.

4.   Heat remaining 1 teaspoon olive oil in a small skillet over medium-low heat, and toast pine nuts for 2 to 3 minutes or until golden brown.

5.   Serve soup hot and garnish with toasted pine nuts.

SERVES 6

2 teaspoons olive oil, divided

1   (1-inch) piece fresh ginger, peeled and minced 1 clove garlic, minced

3/ pound grass-fed, lean beef Sea salt, to taste

2   cups shredded green cabbage 2 cups Beef Stock*

3   cups water

1 cup pearl onions

1   cup julienned carrots 1 bay leaf

2   cups haricots vert

1.   Heat 1 teaspoon olive oil in a Dutch oven over medium heat. Sauté ginger and garlic, stirring constantly to prevent burning.

2.   Trim excess fat from beef and slice as thinly as possible. Add remaining 1 teaspoon olive oil to pot. Add meat and cook until browned, about 2 minutes.

3.   Add cabbage, stock, water, onions, carrots, and bay leaf, and cook 30 minutes.

4.   Add beans to the Dutch oven and cook until beans and carrots are tender, about 10 additional minutes. Remove bay leaf before serving and spoon soup into bowls.

5.   Serve warm.

SERVES 4

soup:

2 teaspoons ghee

1 clove garlic

8 ounces cremini mushrooms, chopped 4 ounces shiitake mushrooms, chopped 4 cups Vegetable Stock*

3 cups water

1/4 cup quinoa

3/4 cup snow peas

pesto:

1/2 cup fresh parsley 1 clove garlic

2 tablespoons olive oil

2   tablespoons lemon juice

1/4   cup raw walnuts 3 tablespoons water Sea salt, to taste

1.   Melt ghee in a stockpot over medium heat and add garlic and mushrooms. Sauté 3 to 4 minutes. Add stock and water, bring to boil, reduce heat to a simmer, and cook 5 minutes.

2.   In the meantime, prepare pesto. In a food processor, combine parsley, garlic, olive oil, lemon juice, walnuts, and water. Season with sea salt, to taste.

3.   Add quinoa to soup and simmer an additional 10 minutes. Add snow peas,

cook 3 minutes, and serve with a dollop of pesto.

SERVES 6

3   tablespoons lemon juice 3 tablespoons olive oil

2 teaspoons dry mustard

1 teaspoon honey or agave Sea salt, to taste

1/ small head of cabbage 2 heads broccoli

1/ cup golden raisins

1/ cup chopped parsley

1. 　　In a large bowl, whisk together lemon juice, olive oil, mustard, honey, and sea salt. Set aside.

2. 　　Remove tough bottoms from cabbage as well as the outer layers. Grate the peeled cabbage into the bowl with the dressing. Cut bottoms and tops off broccoli stems, peel, and grate into same bowl with cabbage. A food processor can also be used for grating.

3. 　　Add raisins and parsley, and toss to mix and coat with dressing.

4. 　　Serve immediately or refrigerate and serve chilled.

SERVES 4

tip: Reserve broccoli tops for a fast recipe: roast at 375 degrees with 2 teaspoons olive oil and a dash of sea salt for 20 minutes.

1 (medium to large) bunch bok choy 2 teaspoons olive oil

1 tablespoon peeled, grated fresh ginger 1 teaspoon minced garlic

1 teaspoon agave Sea salt, to taste

1. 　　Heat grill pan over medium heat.

2. 　　Pull the leaves off the base of the bok choy and slice off the very bottom of the stem to remove any tough pieces. Wash the leaves individually and dry completely on a kitchen towel.

3.   In a small bowl, whisk olive oil, ginger, garlic, and agave. Brush individual bok choy leaves with ginger mixture.

4.   Grill leaves for about 30 to 45 seconds per side, until slightly wilted with golden-brown grill marks. Sprinkle with sea salt, to taste.

5.   Serve warm.

SERVES 4

tip: When purchasing bok choy, look for stalks that are bright white in color with dark-colored greens. Avoid spotted stems and wilted leaves.

1   teaspoon ghee

2   teaspoons olive oil

2 tablespoons finely diced shallots

4 strips nitrate- / preservative-free turkey bacon, diced 4 cups quartered Brussels sprouts

1/ cup Vegetable Stock*

1 tablespoon chopped parsley, for garnish

1.   Heat ghee and olive oil in a large skillet over medium heat. Sauté shallots and turkey bacon until bacon is crispy, about 4 to 5 minutes.

2.   Add Brussels sprouts, and continue to cook for 15 minutes, stirring occasionally to prevent burning. Add raisins and stock, and cook an additional 3 minutes so the raisins can become tender, and the broth can help deglaze the bottom of the pan and add moisture to the sprouts.

3.   Sprouts are done when they can be pierced with a fork but still give moderate resistance. Be careful not to overcook, as they will become mushy and lose a lot of flavor.

4.   Garnish with parsley and serve warm.

SERVES 4

1 tablespoon olive oil

1/2 teaspoon mustard seeds

1/2 teaspoon cumin

1/2 teaspoon almonds

3/4 cup finely diced onion 3 cups diced eggplant

1 cup diced red bell pepper

1/2 teaspoon turmeric

1   teaspoon red chili powder

1.   Heat olive oil in a Dutch oven over medium heat. Add mustard seeds, cumin, and almonds, and cook 30 seconds. Add onions, and cook 5 minutes.

2.   Add eggplant and bell peppers, and cook an additional 15 minutes. Add turmeric, salt, and chili powder, and let cook another 5 minutes.

3.   Serve warm.

SERVES 6

2   teaspoons olive oil

1 cup diced yellow onion 1 clove garlic, minced

1 teaspoon dry mustard 1 teaspoon molasses

1 teaspoon salt

1 teaspoon paprika

1/ teaspoon chili powder

1/ teaspoon cayenne pepper

1   (61/ -oz.) jar whole pimientos, drained

2   (15-oz.) cans navy beans, drained and rinsed

1/ cup Vegetable Stock*

1.   Preheat oven to 375 degrees.

2.   Heat oil in Dutch oven over medium heat. Sauté onion and garlic until translucent and tender, about 5 to 7 minutes. Add mustard, molasses, salt, paprika, chili powder, and cayenne pepper, and cook 1 additional minute.

3.   In a food processor or mini chopper, pulse pimientos until smooth.

4.   Add navy beans, pimiento puree, and stock to pot. Stir to combine.

5.   Cover and bake for 25 minutes until the beans are hot and the sauce is thick.

6.   Serve warm.

SERVES 6

2 teaspoons olive oil 1 teaspoon ghee

1/ cup diced shallots

4 slices nitrate- / preservative-free turkey bacon, finely diced

1/ teaspoon chipotle chili powder 1 bunch collard greens

1	(15-oz.) can cannellini beans, drained and rinsed Sea salt, to taste

1.	Heat olive oil and ghee in a large skillet over medium heat. Add shallots and bacon, and sauté until bacon is crispy, about 4 to 5 minutes. Season with chili powder, add collard greens, and cook 10 to 12 minutes, until collards are tender and wilted.

2.	Add beans, and cook an additional 3 to 4 minutes until warmed through.

3.	Season with sea salt, to taste, and serve warm.

SERVES 4

2	cups cauliflower florets

2 teaspoons olive oil Sea salt, to taste 1 tablespoon ghee

2 cloves garlic, minced

1 cup finely diced white onion 3 tablespoons oat flour

1/2 cup 2 percent cow's milk

3/4 cup Vegetable Stock*

10 cups roughly chopped baby spinach

1.	Preheat oven to 400 degrees.

2.	Toss cauliflower florets with olive oil and sea salt and place on a baking sheet. Bake for 35 minutes, until softened and slightly browned on the bottoms. Remove from oven and set aside.

3.   Melt ghee in a Dutch oven over medium heat. Sauté garlic and onion for 5 to 6 minutes. Add oat flour and stir for about 1 minute just to cook out the taste of the flour. Slowly add milk and stock, whisking continuously to avoid lumps. Continue whisking until mixture becomes the consistency of yogurt, about 5 minutes.

4.   Add spinach, 1/4 at a time, just so it has a chance to cook down and make room for the next batch.

5.   Once all the spinach has been added, toss in roasted cauliflower. Serve warm.

SERVES 4

1 celery root

1   turnip

2   carrots

2 cups cauliflower florets 4 shallots, diced

1   tablespoon olive oil 1 teaspoon sea salt

2   tablespoons chopped fresh sage

1.   Preheat oven to 400 degrees.

2.   Peel celery root, turnip, and carrots. Dice celery, turnip, and carrots into 2- inch pieces.

3.   Toss vegetables, shallots, olive oil, sea salt, and sage in a large bowl until evenly coated.

4.   Pour onto a baking sheet and bake for 55 to 60 minutes, until all vegetables are tender and browned around the edges.

5.   Serve warm.

SERVES 4

2 heads escarole, washed and dried 2 teaspoons olive oil

1/4 teaspoon large-grain sea salt

1.   Preheat oven to 375 degrees.

2.   Trim woody stems off the bottom of escarole and discard, and give the leaves a rough chop. Toss with olive oil and season with sea salt.

3.   Spread escarole evenly across two baking sheets. Bake 10 to 12 minutes, stirring once after 5 minutes. Escarole should be dark green and wilted with

crispy, slightly browned edges.

4.   Serve immediately.

SERVES 4

1 medium bunch mustard greens 2 teaspoons olive oil

1/2 teaspoon sea salt

1/ teaspoon cayenne pepper

1/ cup crumbled feta cheese

1.   Preheat oven to 375 degrees.

2.   Prepare mustard greens by washing and patting dry with a kitchen towel. Remove greens from woody stems and roughly chop or tear into bite-size pieces. Toss with olive oil, sea salt, and cayenne pepper. Spread on a baking sheet and place on the top rack of the oven. Bake 12 minutes, until wilted and slightly crispy around the edges.

3.   Transfer to a serving bowl and add crumbled feta.

4.   Serve warm.

SERVES 4

1   medium eggplant Sea salt, to taste

2   medium red bell peppers

1 bulb fennel

1 large white onion

1 tablespoon olive oil, divided 1 cup peas

1/ cup chopped parsley 2 cloves garlic

1/ cup grated hard goat cheese

1.   Preheat oven to 375 degrees.

2.   Slice eggplant in 1/ -inch-thick rounds, set on a towel, and sprinkle with sea salt to draw out excess moisture. Slice red bell pepper, fennel, and onion in a similar fashion, set aside.

3.   Heat 2 teaspoons olive oil in a large skillet over medium heat. When hot, carefully brown red bell pepper, fennel, and onion in a single layer on the bottom of the pan. Cook vegetables 2 to 3 minutes per side, just to brown. Remove from skillet and set aside.

4.   Pat excess moisture off eggplant slices, and brown in the same skillet, cooking 2 to 3 minutes per side, adding additional oil if necessary. Remove from pan and set aside.

5.   Return skillet to stovetop and increase heat to medium-high. Puree peas in a mini food processor. Add to pan with parsley and garlic, and sauté for 3 to 4 minutes.

6.   In a baking dish, layer red bell pepper and eggplant across the bottom, top with pea mixture and 1/ cup goat cheese. Top with onion, fennel, and remaining cheese.

7.   Bake uncovered for 20 minutes.

8.   Serve warm or let come to room temperature or store in refrigerator, and serve cold.

SERVES 4

1   head broccoli

2   teaspoons olive oil Sea salt, to taste

basil oil:

1 clove garlic

1   cup finely chopped basil 1 tablespoon lemon juice 1 tablespoon olive oil

1–2 tablespoons water

1.   Preheat oven to 375 degrees.

2.   Dice broccoli into bite-size pieces, and toss with olive oil and sea salt. Place on a sheet pan or in a baking dish, and roast for 25 minutes. Broccoli will be deep green with slightly browned edges.

3.   While the broccoli roasts, make basil oil by pureeing garlic, basil, lemon juice, olive oil, and water until thin and runny.

4.   Serve broccoli drizzled with garlic-basil oil.

SERVES 4

2   large sweet potatoes

1   tablespoon plus 2 teaspoons olive oil Sea salt, to taste

1/ teaspoon nutmeg

2   tablespoons fresh sage

1.   Preheat oven to 400 degrees.

2.   Leaving skins on potatoes, cut off tough ends and slice in half lengthwise. Cut in 1/ -inch-thick half-moon shapes and toss with 2 teaspoons olive oil, a dash of sea salt, and nutmeg. Place sweet potato slices in a single layer on a baking sheet, and roast for 25 to 30 minutes or until slightly browned and tender.

3.   During last few minutes of cooking, heat remaining 1 tablespoon olive oil in a small skillet over medium heat. Place sage in pan and fry until crispy, no more than 30 seconds. Remove with a slotted spoon onto a paper towel. Important note: make sure sage is perfectly dry, as wetness on the leaves will splatter the hot oil.

4.   Remove sweet potatoes from oven and serve garnished with crumbled fried sage.

SERVES 4

11/2 cups 2 percent cow's milk 2 sprigs fresh sage

3 egg yolks

1/4 cup brown rice flour

1 tablespoon maple syrup 1 cup sweet potato, baked 1 tablespoon ghee or butter

1 tablespoon fresh sage, finely chopped 1 teaspoon sea salt

6 large egg whites

tip: Egg whites cannot be beaten in a bowl that holds fat, such as plastic. Rather, a glass, copper, or stainless steel bowl will enable to eggs to be beaten into stiff peaks. Water inside the bowl will also prohibit egg whites from stiffening, so make sure to carefully wipe down the inside of the bowl prior to use.

1. Preheat oven to 350 degrees. Grease bottom and sides of 8 (4-oz.) ramekins. Set aside.

2. In a small saucepan, gently warm milk with 2 sprigs of sage for 10 to 12 minutes.

3. While the milk heats, whisk together egg yolks, brown rice flour, and maple syrup. When milk is ready, temper egg yolks by very slowly pouring about 1/2 cup of warm milk into the egg mixture, stirring continuously. Pour the tempered eggs back into the saucepan with the remaining milk. Increase heat to medium, and stir until thickened, 2 to 3 minutes.

4. In a medium bowl, beat baked sweet potato with ghee, finely chopped sage, and salt. When milk mixture has thickened, remove from heat, and whisk in whipped sweet potato until smooth. Cool completely.

5. In a dry, glass, stainless steel, or copper bowl, beat egg whites until they form stiff peaks. Fold egg whites into cooled sweet potato mixture 1⁄3 at a time. Once the egg whites are completely incorporated, spoon batter into prepared ramekins, filling each ramekin 3⁄4 of the way up the sides. Place ramekins in a high-sided baking dish, and place in oven with the oven rack extended out of the oven. Pour

1 inch of hot water into the bottom of the baking dish. Bake soufflés for 55 to 60 minutes or until firm.

6. Serve immediately.

SERVES 6

Rutabaga Smash

2 rutabaga roots

1 head broccoli

1/ cup roughly chopped parsley

1/ cup 2 percent cow's milk 2 cloves garlic, peeled

2   teaspoons ghee or butter Sea salt, to taste

1.   Peel rutabaga and dice in approximately 1-inch pieces to ensure even cooking. Place in a pot with cold, salted water and bring to a boil. Reduce heat, cover, simmer for 35 minutes, or until rutabaga is fork-tender.

2.   Bring a second pot of water to a boil. Trim stems off broccoli and dice into bite-size pieces. Steam 5 to 6 minutes, until bright green and tender. Drain and set aside.

3.   Drain rutabaga and return to pot. Use a potato masher or fork to mash rutabaga, and add parsley, milk, garlic, butter, and salt. Cook 3 to 4 minutes, until butter melts and flavors incorporate, and fold in broccoli.

4.   Serve warm.

SERVES 4

6 cups sliced sweet potatoes 2 teaspoons ghee

1 cup diced onion

1   cup diced green bell pepper 2 links raw turkey sausage

2   teaspoons olive oil Sea salt, to taste

1 tablespoon maple syrup

1.   Slice sweet potatoes into matchsticks, about 2 inches long and 1/ -inch thick. Place sweet potatoes in a large pot of cold water and bring to a boil. As soon as the water boils, drain and spread sweet potatoes out on a baking sheet lined with a kitchen towel, set aside to dry.

2.   Heat 2 teaspoons ghee in a large skillet over medium heat. Sauté onion and bell pepper for 3 to 4 minutes, until tender. Remove turkey sausage from casings and add to onion. Cook for 5 minutes, breaking apart with a flat spatula.

3.   Remove sausage and vegetables from pan and set aside. Add olive oil to skillet, and add sweet potatoes. Do not stir for 2 minutes so potatoes brown on one side. Flip, and let cook undisturbed for 2 to 3 minutes to brown the opposite side. Add sausage and vegetables to the pan with maple syrup and stir gently, just to combine.

4.   Serve hot.

SERVES 6

1   small onion

2   medium carrots

2 stalks celery

1   large parsnip

2   teaspoons olive oil 1 clove garlic, minced

3/4 cup organic sweet potato puree

3   tablespoons chopped sage, divided

1/2 cup Vegetable Stock* Sea salt, to taste

1.   cup Rice Polenta*

1.   Peel and dice onions, carrots, celery, and parsnips into 1/4- to 1/2-inch dice.

2.   Heat olive oil in a large sauté pan over medium heat. Sauté vegetables 5 to 6 minutes until vegetables begin to soften.

3.   Add garlic, sweet potato puree, 2 tablespoons sage, and stock. Season with sea salt, to taste.

4.   Bring to a boil, reduce heat to low, and cook for 20 to 30 minutes, stirring occasionally. Finished ragu should be creamy, and all vegetables should be fork- tender.

5.   Serve warm on top of Rice Polenta, and garnish with remaining sage.

SERVES 4

3/4 cup brown rice 11/2 cups water

2   teaspoons olive oil

1/2 cup diced celery

1 tablespoon chopped fresh sage 1 cup diced shiitake mushrooms

1   cup diced silver dollar mushrooms

1/ cup finely diced shallots 2 cups arugula

2   tablespoons toasted almonds

1.   Cook brown rice in water according to package instructions. Remove from heat and set aside to cool slightly.

2.   Heat olive oil in a medium skillet over medium heat, and sauté celery, sage, mushrooms, and shallots for 3 to 4 minutes, until vegetables just begin to soften.

3.   In a large serving bowl, toss brown rice, sautéed mushroom mixture, arugula, and toasted almonds. The brown rice will be warm and will wilt the arugula slightly.

4.   Serve warm or room temperature.

SERVES 4

2 teaspoons olive oil

1/2 cup finely diced white onion 1 cup forbidden black rice

2 cups Vegetable Stock*

3/4 cup 2 percent cow's milk

1/2 teaspoon sea salt

1.   Heat stock and milk in a small pot over low heat.

2.   Heat olive oil in a Dutch oven over medium heat. Sauté onion and rice for 3

to 4 minutes, stirring constantly.

3.   Add stock mixture, one ladle at a time, to the rice and onions. Season with sea salt. When the liquid is absorbed, add the next ladle. Repeat until all the liquid has been used; this process will take about 45 minutes.

4.   Serve warm.

SERVES 4

1 cup quinoa

1 cup Vegetable Stock* 1 cup water

1 tablespoon fresh rosemary 1 tablespoon fresh thyme

1 tablespoon fresh parsley

1/2 teaspoon lemon zest 2 tablespoons flaxseeds

1/ cup crumbled feta cheese

1. Combine quinoa, stock, and water in a pot. Bring to a boil, reduce heat, and simmer for 10 to 12 minutes. When quinoa is done, all the water will be absorbed, and quinoa will be soft and tender.

2. Fluff cooked quinoa with a fork, and toss with remaining ingredients. Serve warm.

SERVES 4

1 small head broccoli 1 bunch broccolini

1 (4-inch) piece lemongrass

1   cup quinoa

2   cups water

2 teaspoons olive oil

1   red bell pepper, diced 1 tablespoon lemon zest Sea salt, to taste

1. Bring a large pot of water to a boil. Chop broccoli and broccolini into bite- size pieces, drop into water, and cook for 3 minutes. Remove with a slotted spoon, and place in an ice bath to stop the cooking process. Drain and set aside on a kitchen towel.

2. Bruise lemongrass by hammering with the back of your knife, just until aromatic. Bring quinoa and water to a boil with a pinch of salt, and reduce heat to simmer. Add lemongrass to the quinoa, and let cook 12 minutes.

3.   Heat olive oil in a large skillet over medium heat, and sauté bell pepper for 3 to 4 minutes. Add broccoli and broccolini, and sauté an additional 2 to 3 minutes. Vegetables should be crisp-tender and remain brightly colored when finished cooking. Remove lemongrass from cooked quinoa. Toss vegetables with quinoa and lemon zest, adding sea salt, to taste.

Chapter 6: Four-Week Meal Planner

Week 1

Sunday

BREAKFAST: Pear-Rosemary Bread NS with sliced banana and raw walnuts LUNCH: Ratatouille NS with sliced mozzarella cheese SNACK: Cucumber slices with Curried Egg Salad NS

DINNER: Chili, Sans Tomatoes

Monday

BREAKFAST: Blackstrap-Cherry Rice Granola NS, rice cereal, and almond milk with green tea and fresh blueberries LUNCH: Leftover Chili, Sans Tomatoes with mixed green salad dressed with lemon and olive oil

SNACK: Pear and Apple Chips and Spicy Rosemary-Nut Mix NS DINNER: Lemon-Ginger Salmon NS with Brown Rice Salad NS

Tuesday

BREAKFAST: Scrambled Eggs with Blueberry-Macadamia Muffins and green tea LUNCH: Raw Kale Salad with Zesty Lime Dressing NS and leftover Lemon-Ginger Salmon NS

SNACK: Flax Crackers NS and Summer Squash Salsa NS

DINNER: Crispy-Coated Turkey Tenders with Apricot Dipping Sauce and Sweet Potato Ragu NS

Wednesday

BREAKFAST: Homemade Turkey Breakfast Sausage NS with green tea and fresh raspberries LUNCH: Raw Kale Salad with Zesty Lime Dressing NS and leftover Crispy-Coated Turkey Tenders with Apricot Dipping Sauce

SNACK: Pear and Apple Chips and Spicy Rosemary-Nut Mix NS DINNER: Grilled Radicchio and Walnut-Spinach Pesto NS

Thursday

BREAKFAST: Blueberry-Macadamia Muffins with leftover Homemade

Turkey Breakfast Sausage NS and green tea LUNCH: Greens and Beans Salad NS with walnuts and crumbled feta SNACK: Protein Blend™ Powder—Type B drink DINNER: Tangy Pineapple and Beef Kabobs NS with Roasted Autumn Roots NS

Friday

BREAKFAST: Quinoa Muesli, banana slices, blueberries, and green tea LUNCH:

Leftover Greens and Beans Salad NS with leftover Tangy Pineapple and Beef Kabobs NS

SNACK: Carob–Walnut Butter–Stuffed Figs NS

DINNER: Mac and Cheese with Roasted Vegetables NS and Garlic–Creamed Spinach with Roasted Cauliflower NS

Saturday

BREAKFAST: Swiss Chard and Cremini Frittata NS with green tea and pineapple LUNCH: 1/2 Bacon Grilled Cheese NS with Roasted Parsnip Soup

NS

SNACK: Almond-Butter Rice Cakes with Mini Chips NS
DINNER: Seafood Paella NS

Week 2

Sunday

BREAKFAST: Cherry Scones NS with almond butter and green tea LUNCH:

Kidney Bean Stew SNACK: Grilled Pineapple with Chocolate Syrup

DINNER: Moroccan Lamb Tagine

Monday

BREAKFAST: Breakfast Egg Salad NS with green tea LUNCH: Mint and Red Pepper Tabbouleh NS with leftover Moroccan Lamb Tagine SNACK: Homemade Applesauce DINNER: Shredded Turkey Bake

Tuesday

BREAKFAST: Quinoa Muesli with sliced bananas and fresh blueberries LUNCH: Leftover Shredded Turkey Bake with mixed greens dressed in olive oil and lemon SNACK: Grilled Pineapple with Chocolate Syrup DINNER: Beef and Shredded Cabbage Soup NS and Red Quinoa- Mushroom Casserole with Fried Egg NS

Wednesday

BREAKFAST: Swiss Chard and Cremini Frittata NS with sliced pineapple and green tea LUNCH: Leftover Red Quinoa–Mushroom Casserole with Fried Egg NS

SNACK: Cheese Toast NS

DINNER: Parchment-Baked Snapper NS

Thursday

BREAKFAST: Broccoli-Feta Frittata NS with green tea LUNCH: Navy Bean Hummus and Feta Sandwich NS

SNACK: Homemade Applesauce DINNER: Rice and Bean Loaf NS with Spicy Collards NS and Baked Beans NS

Friday

BREAKFAST: Nut Butter–Granola Boats NS with green tea LUNCH: Leftover

Rice and Bean Loaf NS sandwiches SNACK: Protein Blend™ Powder— Type B drink DINNER: Spicy Seafood Stew NS

Saturday

BREAKFAST: Spelt Pancakes NS with scrambled eggs and green tea LUNCH:

Salmon-Filled Radicchio Cups NS SNACK: Crispy Spring Vegetable Cakes NS

DINNER: Sweet Potato Gnocchi with Basil-Cranberry Sauce NS with grilled turkey cutlets

Week 3
Sunday

BREAKFAST: Pear-Rosemary Bread NS with a poached egg and green tea

LUNCH: Fish Fillet Sandwich NS

SNACK: Crudités and Creamy Goat Cheese Dip NS

DINNER: Turkey Mole Drumsticks with Whipped Sweet Potato Soufflé and Broccoli and Cabbage Slaw with Raisins NS

Monday

BREAKFAST: Creamy Banana–Nut Butter Smoothie NS and green tea LUNCH:

Leftover Turkey Mole Drumsticks and Broccoli and Cabbage Slaw with Raisins NS

SNACK: Unibar® Protein Bar DINNER: Salmon and Bean Cakes with Cilantro- Cream Sauce NS and Spicy Roasted Mustard Greens with Feta NS

Tuesday

BREAKFAST: Pear-Rosemary Bread NS with scrambled eggs and green tea

LUNCH: Leftover Salmon and Bean Cakes with Cilantro-Cream Sauce NS

and romaine lettuce dressed in lemon and olive oil SNACK: Marinated Mozzarella Balls NS with Flax Crackers NS

DINNER: Hearty Slow-Cooker Turkey Stew NS with Sweet-and-Salty Brussels

NS

Wednesday

BREAKFAST: Turkey Bacon–Spinach Squares NS and green tea LUNCH:

Leftover Hearty Slow-Cooker Turkey Stew NS

SNACK: Unibar® Protein Bar DINNER: Mushroom Soup with Parsley Pesto NS

with Green Tea–Poached Turkey Tenderloins NS

Thursday

BREAKFAST: Blackstrap-Cherry Rice Granola NS and yogurt with green tea and fresh blueberries LUNCH: Shredded leftover Green Tea–Poached Turkey Tenderloins NS with cranberries and walnuts over spinach greens

with olive oil and lemon SNACK: Marinated Mozzarella Balls NS with Flax Crackers NS

DINNER: Fig-Stuffed Turkey Breasts with Roasted Sweet Potatoes with Fried Sage NS

Friday

BREAKFAST: Homemade Turkey Breakfast Sausage NS with green tea and fresh raspberries LUNCH: Leftover Fig-Stuffed Turkey Breasts with Roasted Sweet Potatoes with Fried Sage NS over Raw Kale Salad with Zesty Lime Dressing NS

SNACK: Unibar® Protein Bar DINNER: Spiced Lamb with Wild Mushrooms

NS with Broccoli–Northern Bean Soup NS

Saturday

BREAKFAST: Spinach-Pepper Soufflé NS and green tea LUNCH: Crunchy Vegetable Spring Rolls with Sweet Cherry Dip NS

SNACK: Farmer Cheese and Beet-Endive Cups NS DINNER: Spring Pesto Pasta NS with grilled halibut

Week 4

Sunday

BREAKFAST: Savory Herb and Cheese Bread Pudding NS LUNCH: Navy Bean Hummus and Feta Sandwich NS

SNACK: Tropical Fruit Salad with Mint and Lime Dressing NS DINNER: Sweet Potato Shepherd's Pie NS with Roasted Escarole NS

Monday

BREAKFAST: Maple-Sausage Scramble NS and green tea LUNCH: Leftover Sweet Potato Shepherd's Pie NS

SNACK: Roasted Cauliflower Bruschetta NS

DINNER: Baked Mahimahi with Crunchy Fennel Salad NS and Herbed Quinoa

NS

Tuesday

BREAKFAST: Sweet Potato Muffins with Carob Drizzle with almond butter and green tea LUNCH: Baked Falafel NS and Roasted-Eggplant Greek Salad NS

SNACK: Tropical Fruit Salad with Mint and Lime Dressing NS

DINNER: Greek Lamb Burgers NS and Broccolini with Crispy Walnut Bacon

NS

Wednesday

BREAKFAST: Nut Butter–Granola Boats NS with yogurt and green tea LUNCH:

Leftover Broccolini with Crispy Walnut Bacon NS wrapped in Boston Bibb lettuce with goat cheese SNACK: Crudités and Navy Bean Hummus

NS

DINNER: Turkey-Ginger Stir-Fry NS with Carrot-Ginger Soup NS

Thursday

BREAKFAST: Breakfast Egg Salad NS with green tea LUNCH: Leftover Carrot- Ginger Soup NS and 1/2 Bacon Grilled Cheese NS

SNACK: Roasted Cauliflower Bruschetta NS

DINNER: Pasta Carbonara with Asparagus NS with Greens and Beans Salad NS

Friday

BREAKFAST: Sweet Potato Muffins with Carob Drizzle with almond butter and green tea LUNCH: Leftover Greens and Beans Salad NS with walnuts and fresh mozzarella SNACK: Crudités and Creamy Goat Cheese Dip NS

DINNER: Fish Tacos with Bean and Crunchy Fennel Slaw NS

Saturday

BREAKFAST: Oat Crêpes and green tea LUNCH: Melted Mozzarella–Onion Soup NS

SNACK: Baked Grapefruit DINNER: Turkey Pot Pie with Crunchy Topping NS

Tracking Your Progress This is an additional log to help you focus on your goals.

Shopping List Make your shopping trip easy with this list of Beneficial

foods for your type.

Chapter 7: TYPE B SHOPPING LIST

- **Produce:**
- Beets Broccoli Cabbage Carrots Eggplant Ginger Kale Peppers
- Sweet potatoes Bananas Cranberries Grapes
- Pineapple Watermelon Baking:
- Brown rice flour Millet flour Oat flour Spelt flour Baking powder Sea salt Agave
- Molasses

- Dairy:
- Butter
- Cottage cheese Cow's milk Eggs
- Feta cheese Goat cheese Mozzarella Ricotta Yogurt
- Meat/Seafood:
- Cod Flounder Halibut Lamb Mahimahi Salmon Turkey Venison
- Miscellaneous:
- Olive oil Almonds Almond butter Walnuts
- Kidney beans Navy beans Oat bread Spelt bread Cayenne pepper Parsley Ginger tea Green tea Peppermint tea Please note: This shopping list only
- highlights the most frequently used Beneficial and some Neutral foods for Type B. For a complete list of Beneficials, Neutrals, and Avoids, refer to Eat Right 4 Your Type, the Blood Type B Food, Beverage, and

CPSIA information can be obtained
at www.ICGtesting.com
Printed in the USA
LVHW011345240921
698652LV00023B/1765